DIAGNOSTIC PICTURE TESTS IN

Gastroenterology

Miles C. Allison, MD, MRCP
Gastroenterology Department
Royal Infirmary
Glasgow
Scotland

Part 2 of 2

Presented as a service by

Glaxo Pharmaceuticals™
DIVISION OF GLAXO INC.
Research Triangle Park, NC 27709

Wolfe Publishing Ltd

FOREWORD

In this second volume, Dr Miles Allison has prepared yet another remarkable collection of images relating to gastrointestinal disease. Classical gastroenterology has relatively few physical signs amenable to photography—however, gastroenterology in the 1990s involves not only the physical signs on the skin and various orifices, but also the results of endoscopy, histology, surgery, and modern radiology. Dr Allison has posed tantalizing questions concerning each illustration, and the reader can turn to the back of the book for confirmation of the correct answer or a succinct explanation.

This book should be of value and interest to anyone who sees patients with gastrointestinal disease—from the clinical medical student to the consultant gastroenterologist.

Roy Pounder
Academic Department of Medicine
Royal Free Hospital School of Medicine
London, England

Published by Wolfe Publishing Ltd, 1991
Printed by BPCC Hazell Books Ltd, Aylesbury, England.
ISBN 0-7234-1500-5

This edition is published for Glaxo Pharmaceuticals, a division of Glaxo Inc., by Wolfe Publishing Ltd, London, UK, in association with:
Caduceus Medical Publishers Inc.
Patterson, NY, USA

For full details of Wolfe titles, please write to
Wolfe Publishing Ltd, Brook House, 2–16 Torrington Place,
London WC1E 7LT, England.

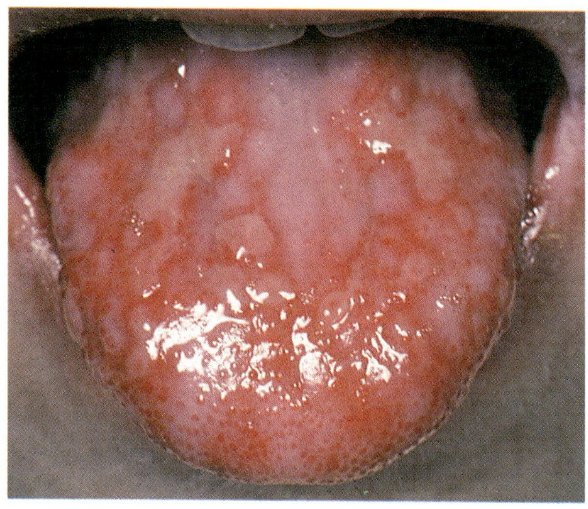

94

94, 95 A 22-year-old man underwent chemotherapy and bone-marrow transplantation for acute leukaemia. This was complicated by septicaemia due to *Candida albicans* for which he received intravenous amphotericin. He was subsequently referred with diarrhoea, weight loss and a sore tongue. His nail changes are shown in **95**.

(a) What is the likely cause of his gastrointestinal symptoms?

(b) How may this be confirmed?

(c) What other causes of diarrhoea should be excluded?

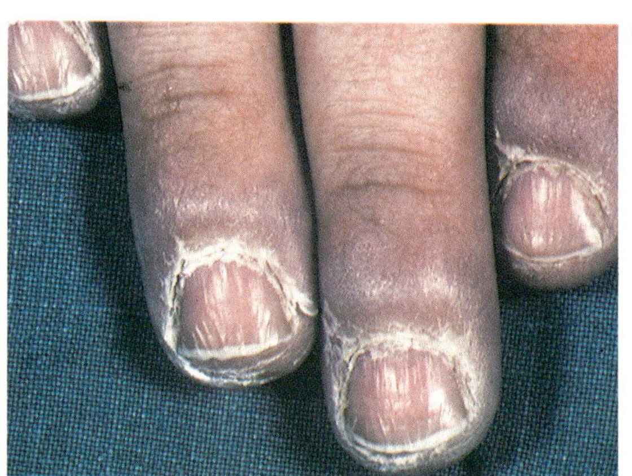

95

96

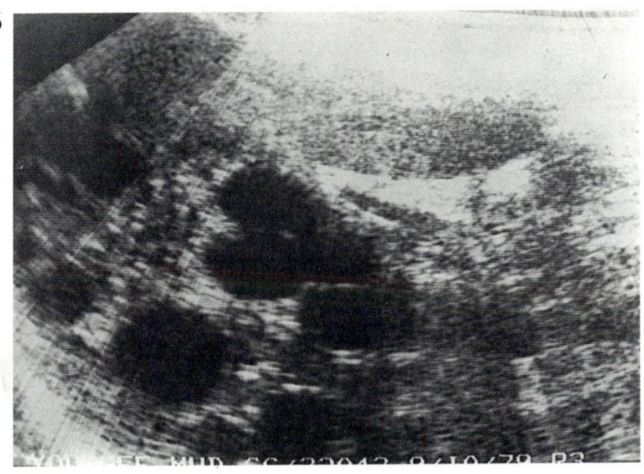

96 A 45-year-old Greek export manager presented with right upper quadrant pain. A liver ultrasound was performed.
(a) What abnormality is demonstrated?
(b) What is the most likely diagnosis?
(c) How may this diagnosis be confirmed?

97 A 44-year-old man presented with drowsiness, constipation and large bilateral pleural effusions. On examination, he was jaundiced and had tense ascites. He was found to be hypoxic.
(a) Give two possible mechanisms for the abnormalities seen here.
(b) Give three possible mechanisms for his hypoxia.

97

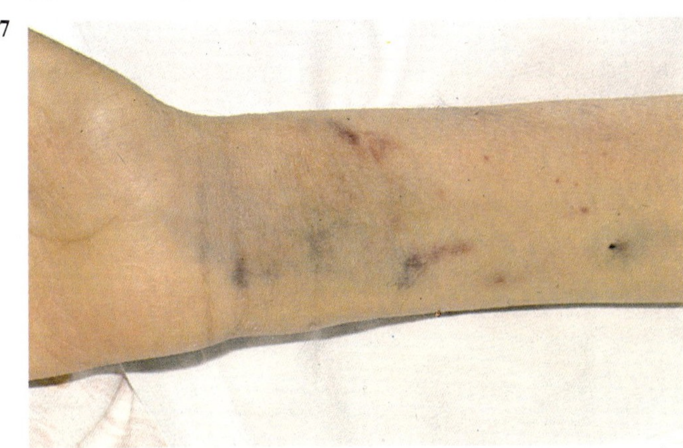

98 A 92-year-old man was referred with diarrhoea and abdominal distension.

(a) What is the diagnosis?

(b) What other disease may be associated?

(c) What is the standard treatment?

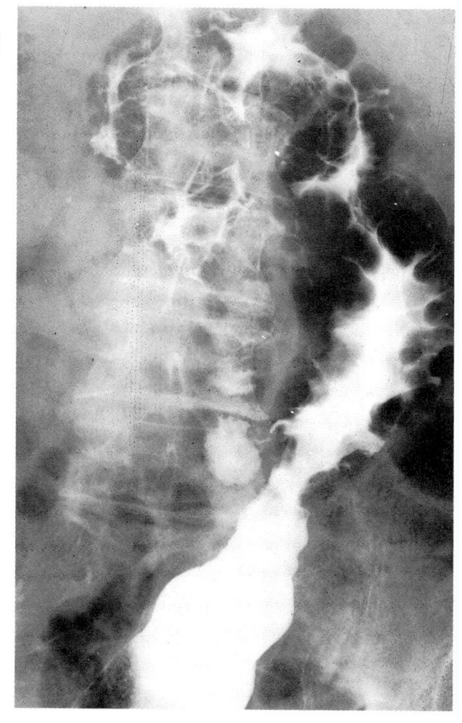

98

99 A 52-year-old man underwent investigation for chronic upper abdominal pain.

(a) What abnormality is seen on this ERCP?

(b) What is the diagnosis?

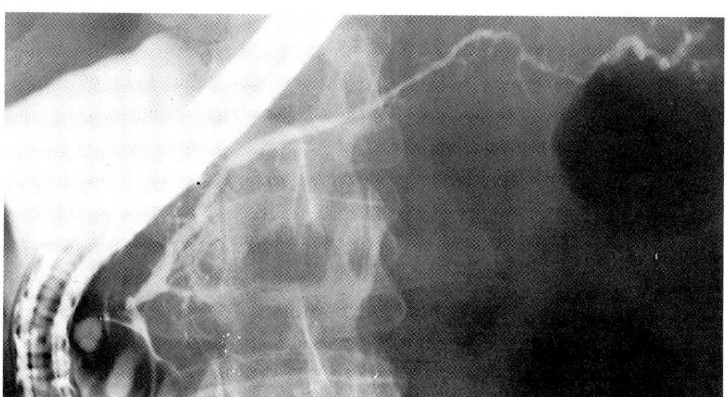

99

100

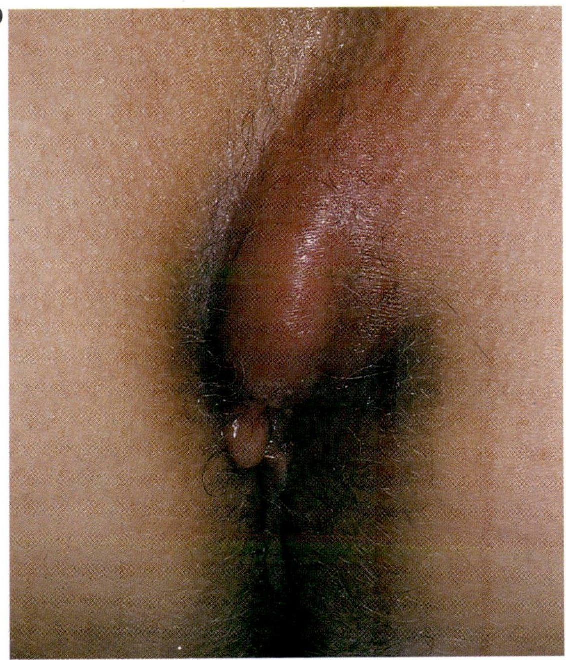

100 A 35-year-old woman with quiescent Crohn's disease developed acute pain above the anus.
(a) What is this lesion?
(b) How is this managed?

101

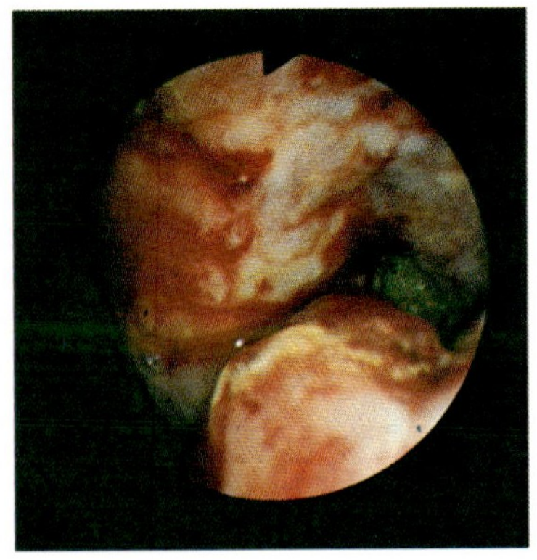

101 A 66-year-old woman underwent upper gastrointestinal endoscopy for investigation of vomiting and weight loss.
(a) What gastric abnormality is shown?
(b) What confirmatory investigation should be performed?
(c) Give three well recognised predisposing factors.

102 A 65-year-old woman presented with fever, rigors and dark urine.
(a) What is the most likely cause of this appearance on barium meal?
(b) What complication has developed?
(c) Give two possible explanations for this complication.

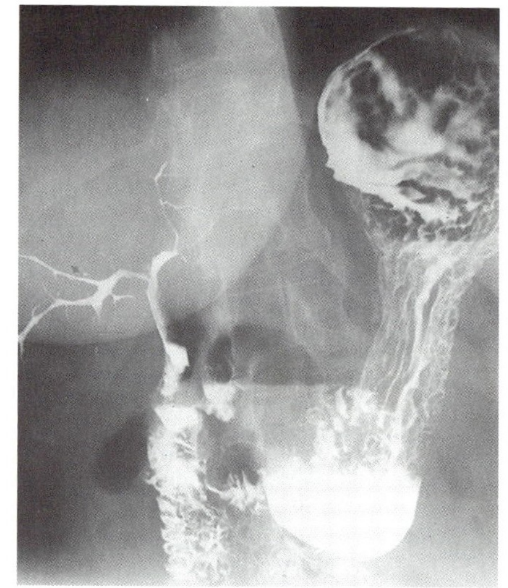

102

103 This 62-year-old man presented with a three-month history of right upper quadrant pain and weight loss. His liver was enlarged five finger-breadths below the right costal margin and was tender.
(a) What is the most likely diagnosis?
(b) Give two non-invasive investigations which may be helpful in confirming the diagnosis.

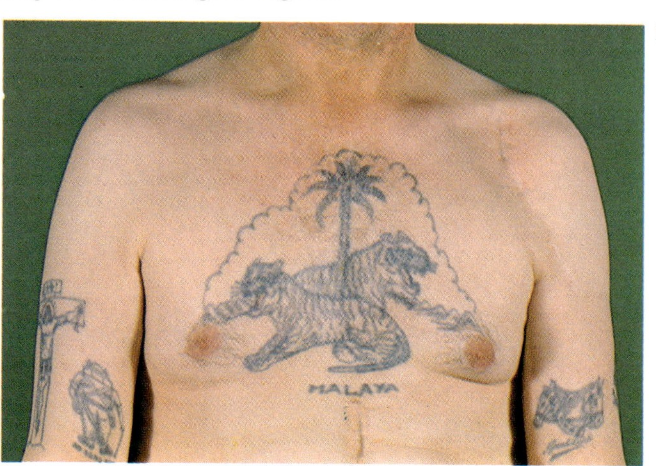

103

104

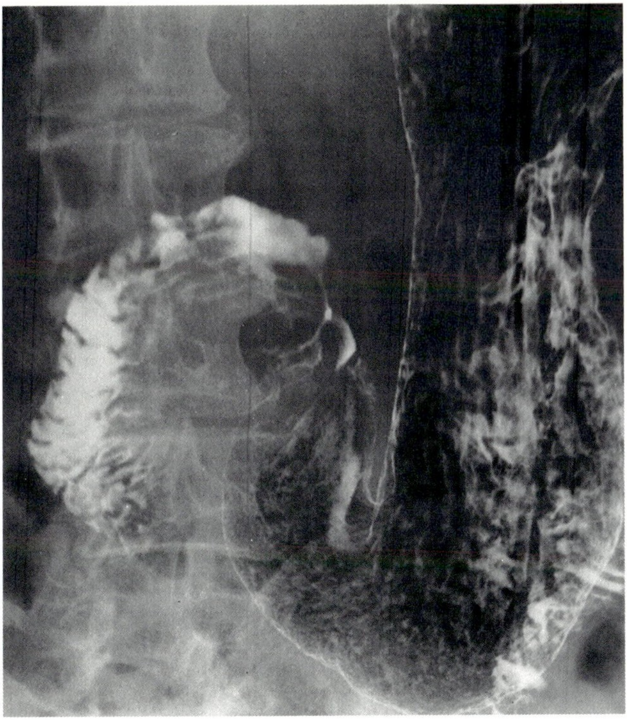

104 A 34-year-old man underwent a barium meal following the passage of a melaena stool.
(a) Describe the radiological abnormality.
(b) What is the diagnosis?

105

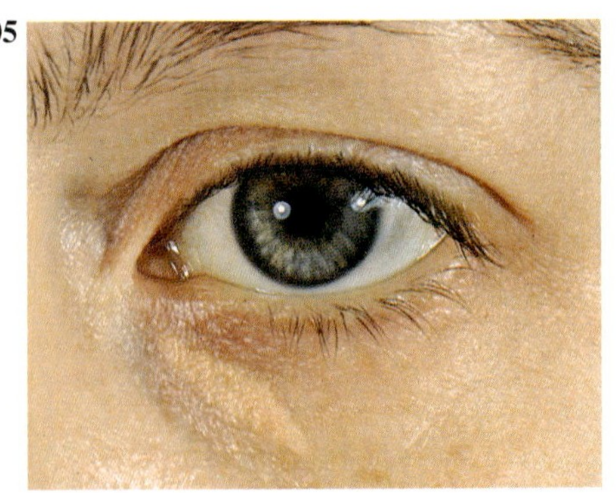

105 A 38-year-old woman complained of generalised itching. There was a history of dry eyes and recurrent urinary tract infections.
(a) What is the most likely diagnosis?
(b) Give three investigations which will confirm the diagnosis.

106 A 34-year-old woman was admitted to an infectious disease unit with a three-week history of bloodstained diarrhoea. She had been treated for a chest infection one month previously, but had otherwise been well. Routine stool microscopy and culture were negative. She was fasted and given intravenous fluids. Three days later she felt considerably better, her stool frequency had reduced, but her temperature had not returned to normal.

(a) What is the most likely diagnosis?
(b) What complication has developed?
(c) Which three further investigations should have been done on this patient?

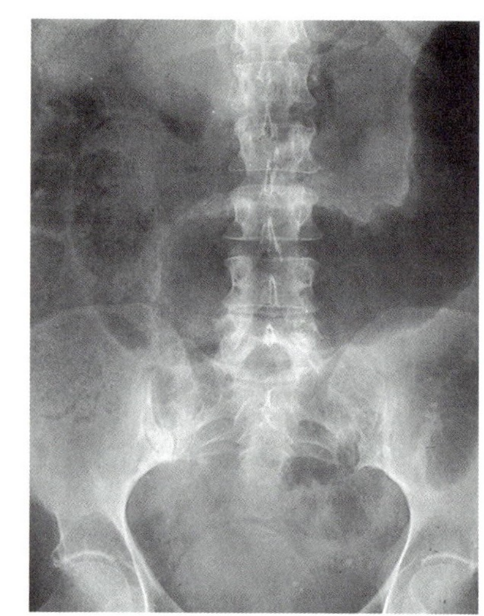

106

107 A 50-year-old man presented with melaena and shock. Several of these lesions were present on the limbs and trunk.

(a) What is the diagnosis?
(b) What other gastrointestinal complication may occur?

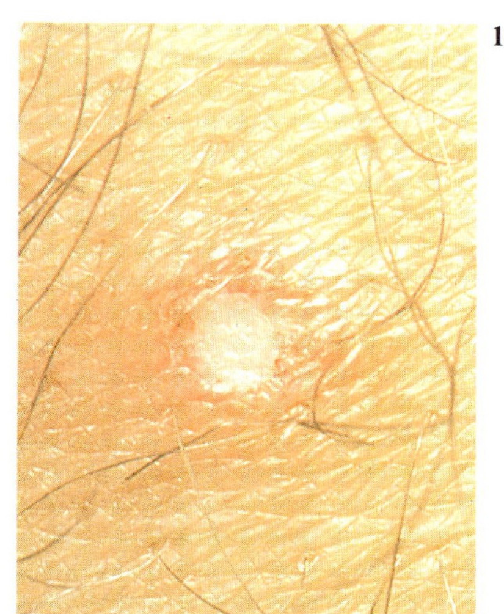

107

108

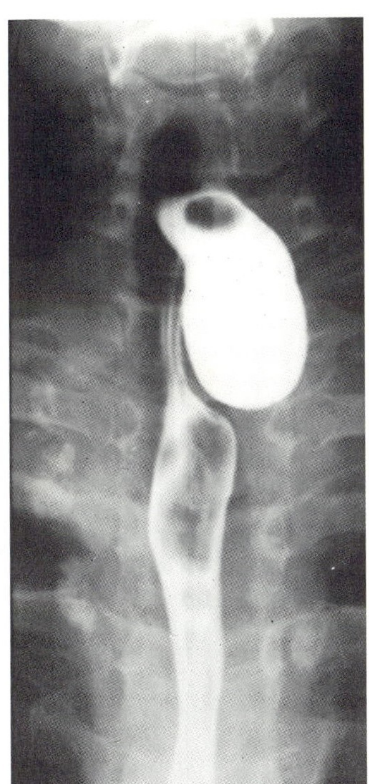

108 This barium swallow was performed in a 69-year-old woman who had been experiencing regurgitation after meals.
(a) What abnormality is seen?
(b) What important complication may occur?
(c) Should endoscopy be performed?
(d) How should she be treated?

109 A 28-year-old man attended for a routine dental check-up. He had developed a sore mouth and lost 3 kg in weight recently, but had no other symptoms.
(a) What is the diagnosis?
(b) What is the most likely predisposing factor in this case?
(c) Give three other predisposing factors for this condition.

109

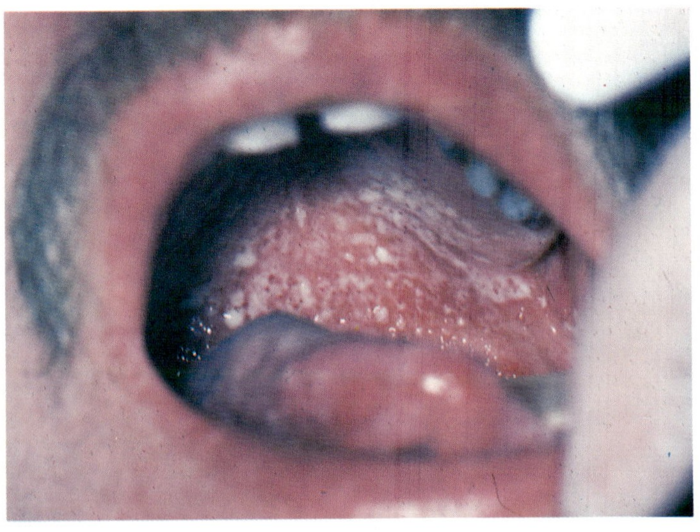

110 A 21-year-old woman developed pain in her left knee. On examination, there was no joint tenderness, but a small effusion was present. On direct questioning, she admitted to occasional urgency of defaecation and liquid stools since starting the oral contraceptive pill six months previously. Barium enema was normal. This photograph was taken during colonoscopy.
(a) What term is given to this endoscopic appearance?
(b) What is the most likely diagnosis?
(c) What is the cause of the joint pain?

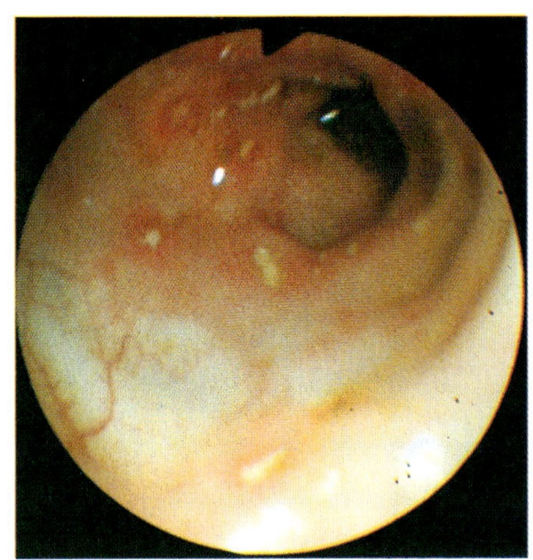

110

111 A 71-year-old woman gave a three-week history of jaundice, pale stools, dark urine and weight loss. Ultrasound demonstrated a dilated biliary tree and several stones in the gall bladder. An ERCP was performed.
(a) What is the reason for her jaundice?
(b) Give two possible alternatives for treatment.

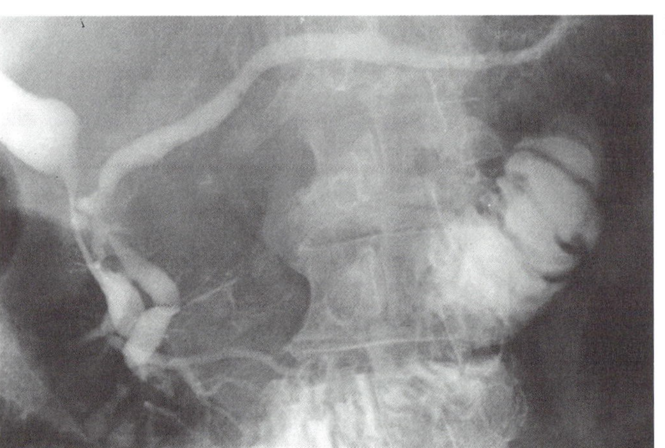

111

112

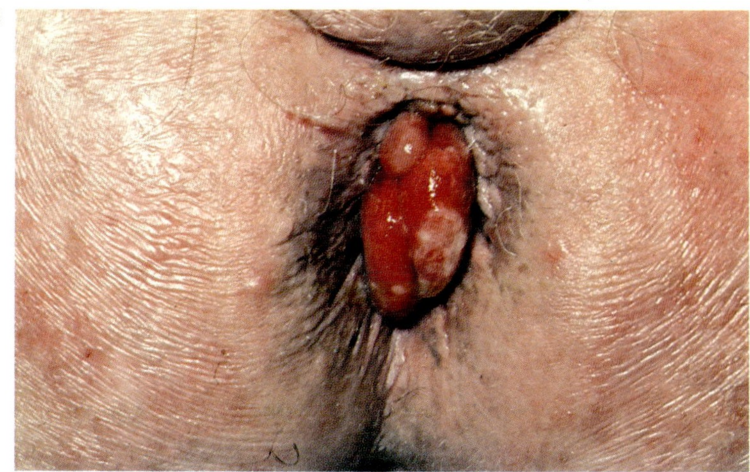

112 A 64-year-old man was referred to the surgical clinic with pruritus ani and perianal discharge.

(a) What is the diagnosis?
(b) Which virus has recently been linked with this condition?
(c) How should he be managed?

113

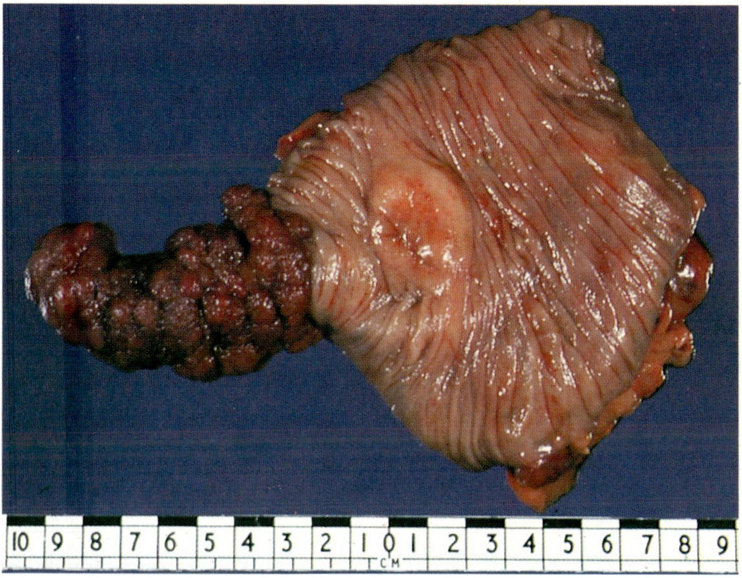

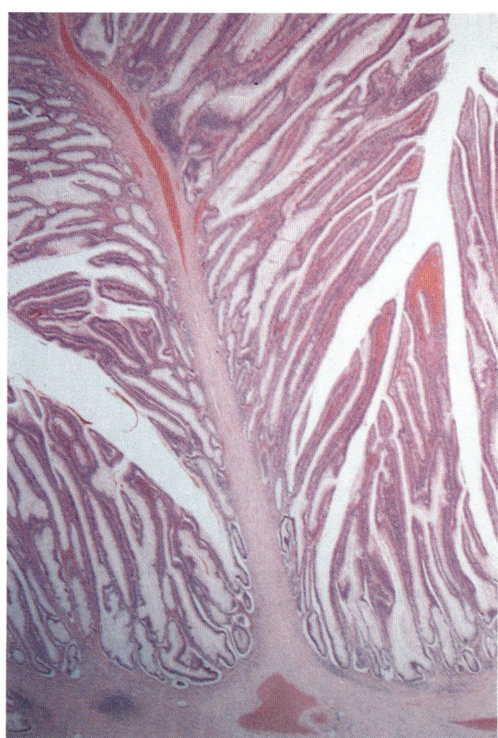

114

113, 114 An 81-year-old man presented with watery diarrhoea and dehydration. The stool was positive for occult blood. The colonic lesion in **113** was resected and its histological appearance is shown in **114**.

(a) What is the lesion?

(b) What electrolyte disturbance may have occurred in this patient?

115

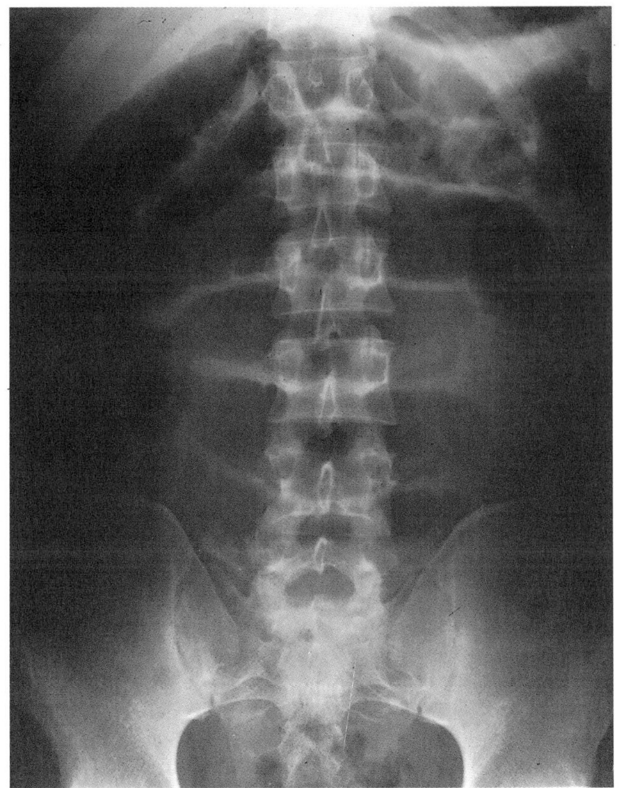

115 A 64-year-old man was admitted as an emergency with abdominal pain and vomiting.
(a) What abnormality is shown on this plain abdominal radiograph?
(b) What are the two commonest causes of this appearance?

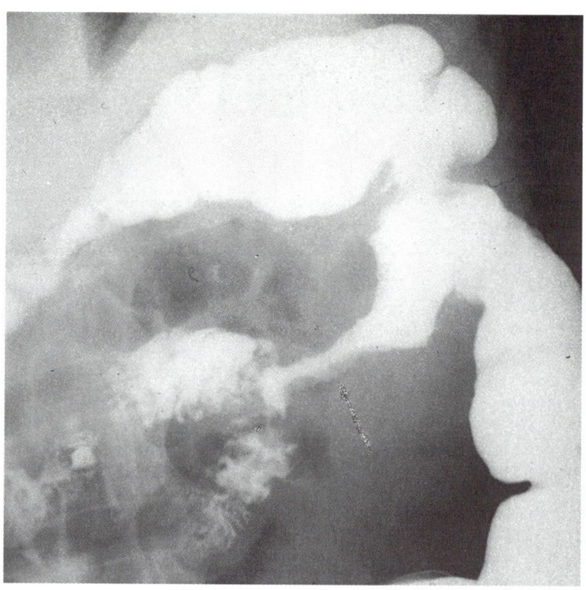

116

116 A barium enema was performed in a 62-year-old man with abrupt onset of diarrhoea and loss of 5 kg in weight.
(a) What abnormality has been demonstrated?
(b) What is the most likely underlying cause?
(c) What two mechanisms contributed to the diarrhoea in this patient?

117 A 38-year-old woman who lived alone was found lying on the floor unconscious. She was markedly dehydrated, hypotensive, jaundiced and had a distended abdomen due to ascites. Bowel sounds were absent.
(a) What is the name given to the physical sign seen here?
(b) What is the diagnosis?
(c) What has caused this appearance to develop?

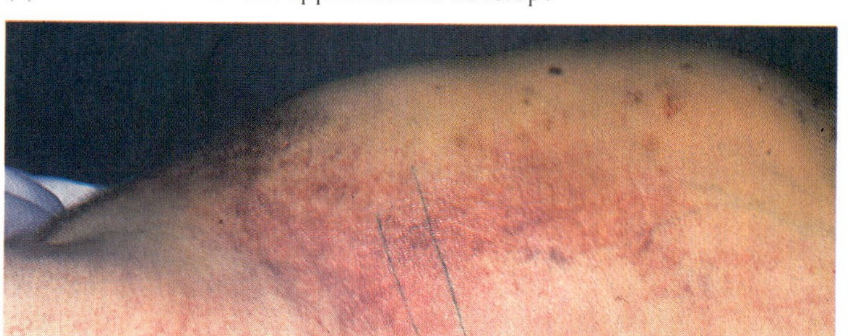

117

118

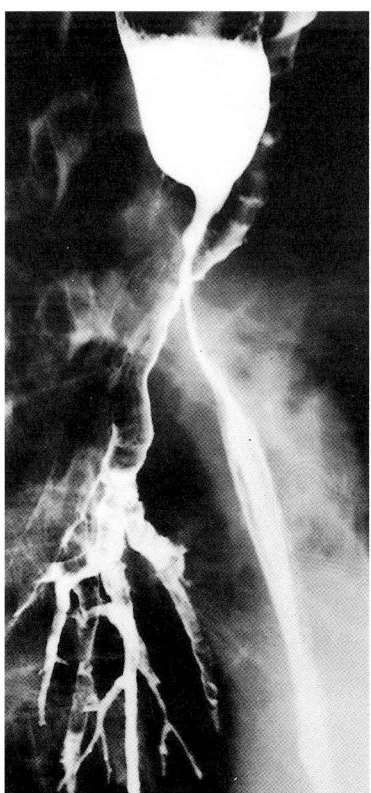

119

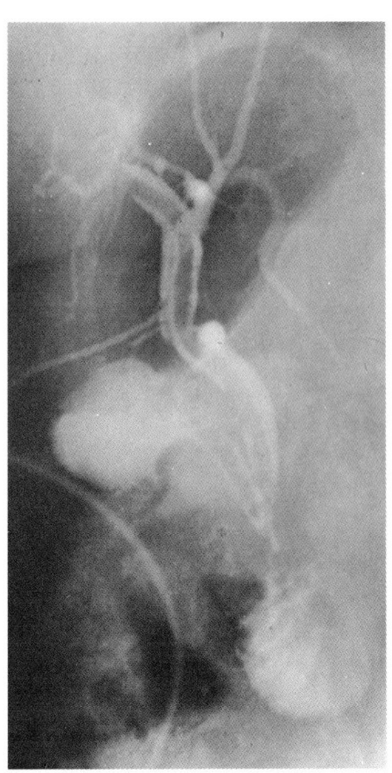

118 A 72-year-old man presented with dysphagia and a cough with purulent sputum. A barium swallow was performed.
(a) What is the most likely diagnosis?
(b) What complication has developed?
(c) How would the patient be best managed?

119 A 35-year-old mentally retarded woman developed right upper quadrant pain and dark urine. Oral cholecystography failed to opacify the gall bladder, and she proceeded to cholecystectomy on the presumption that gallstones were present. This investigation was performed post-operatively.
(a) What investigation is being performed?
(b) What abnormality has been demonstrated?
(c) Give three possible approaches to treatment.

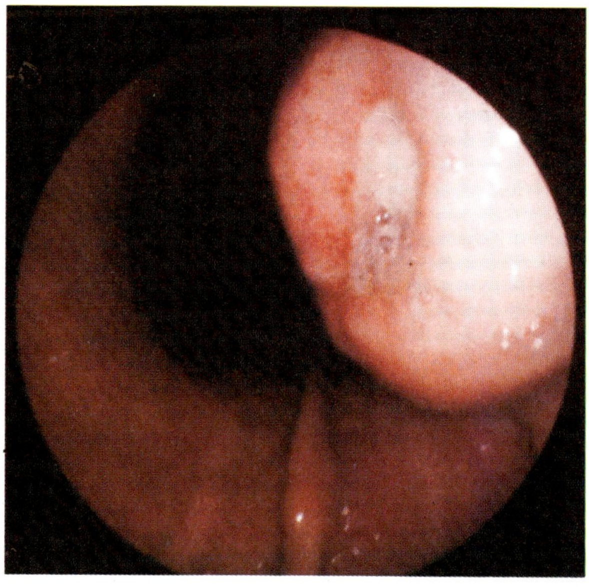

120

120 A 68-year-old woman underwent endoscopic investigation following two episodes of haematemesis and melaena within the previous month.
(a) What is the diagnosis?
(b) What rare complication may develop within these lesions?
(c) What treatment would you recommend?

121 A 32-year-old man with a history of intravenous drug abuse developed weight loss, high fever and painless haematuria. He was known to be positive for the hepatitis B surface antigen.
(a) What is the abnormality seen here?
(b) Where else would you look for similar lesions?
(c) Give two possible diagnoses.

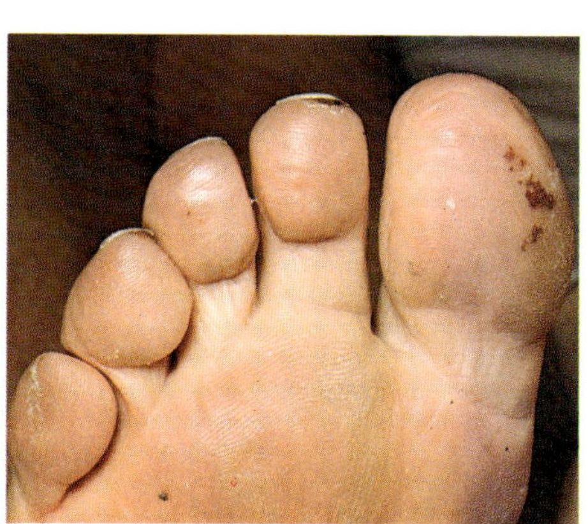

121

122

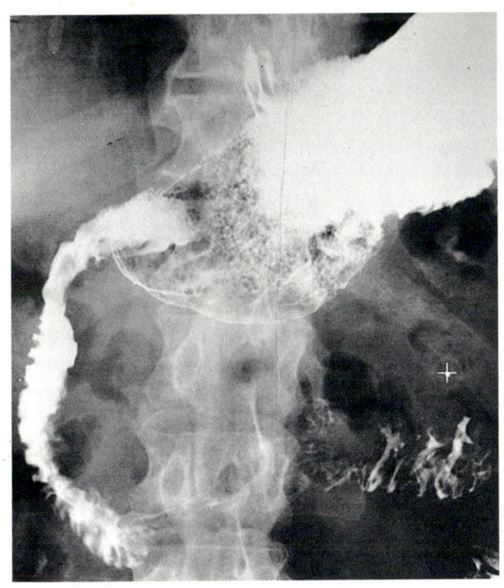

122 A 72-year-old woman underwent a barium meal examination for the investigation of recent weight loss and epigastric pain.
(a) What abnormality is demonstrated?
(b) What is the most likely diagnosis?

123

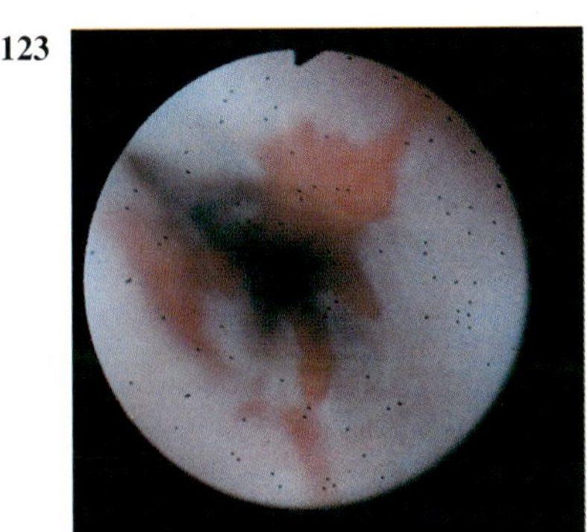

123 This endoscopic photograph was taken with the tip of the endoscope positioned in the oesophagus 28 cm from the incisor teeth.
(a) What feature is demonstrated?
(b) What is the diagnosis?
(c) Give three late complications which may develop in this patient.

124

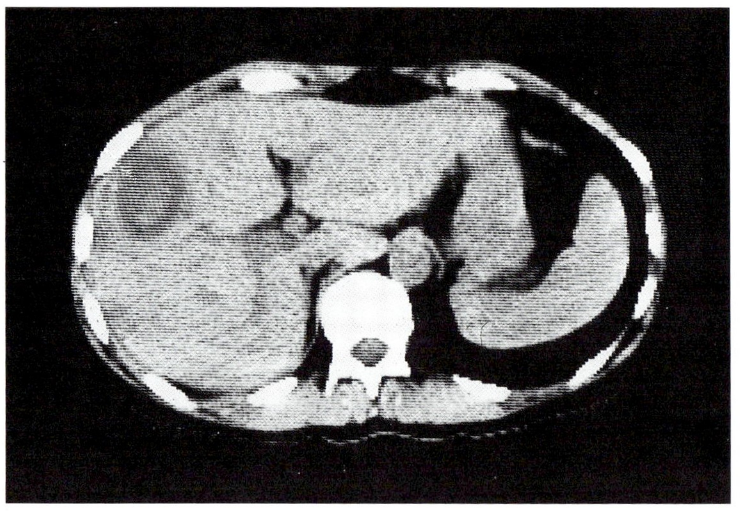

124 A 34-year-old woman presented with right upper quadrant pain and fever. She had returned from a holiday in Kenya two months previously and had been a regular user of the oral contraceptive pill for seven years.
(a) What is the most likely diagnosis?
(b) Give two investigations which may be helpful in confirming the diagnosis.
(c) What is the treatment of choice?

125

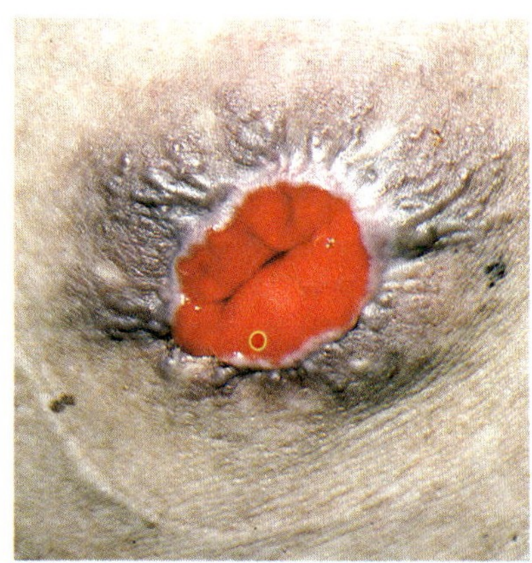

125 A 56-year-old man had undergone panproctocolectomy and ileostomy for ulcerative colitis five years previously. He complained of recurrent haemorrhage from around the stoma site.
(a) What is the cause of the recurrent haemorrhage?
(b) What is the probable underlying explanation for the development of this condition?

126

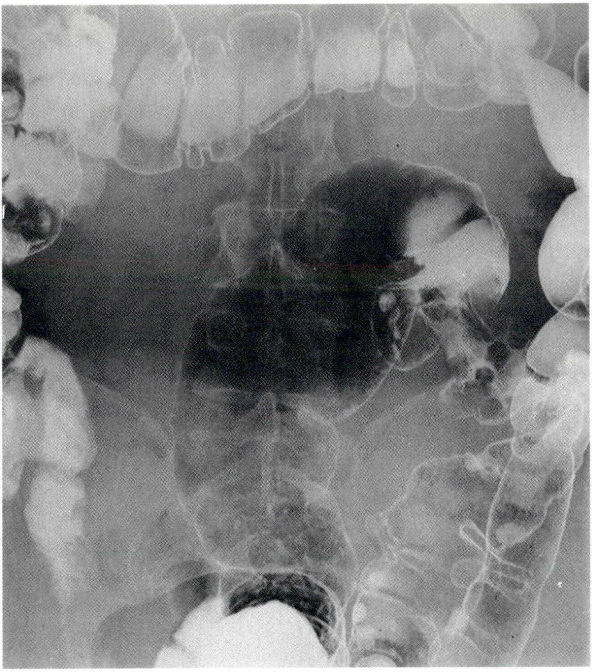

126 A 50-year-old man presented with an alteration in bowel habit.
(a) What is the diagnosis?
(b) What two roles may colonoscopy play in this patient?

127

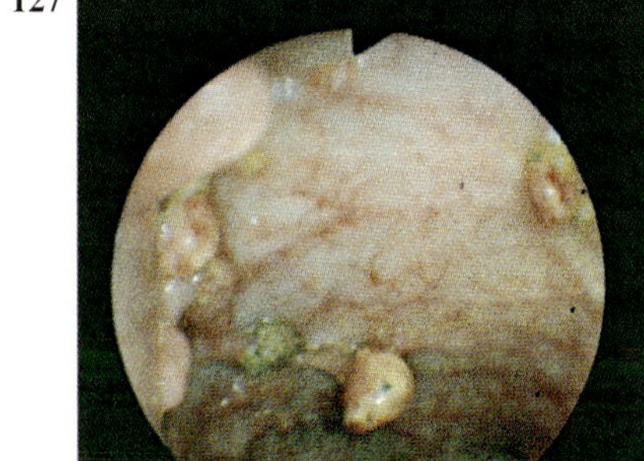

127 This view was obtained in the distal sigmoid colon in a 54-year-old woman with a 20-year history of extensive ulcerative colitis.
(a) What abnormality is shown?
(b) How does this finding affect management of the patient?
(c) Comment on the degree of activity of the colitis.

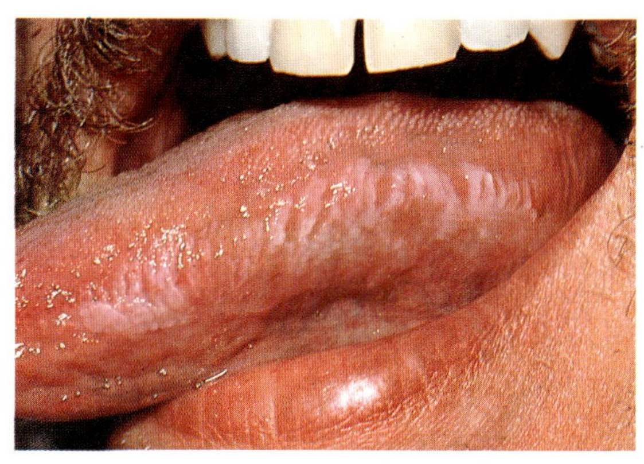

128

128, 129 A 28-year-old man presented with abdominal pain, diarrhoea and weight loss. He was an unmarried travelling salesman who regularly visited Africa. A smear of a formol-ether stool concentrate is illustrated in **129**.

(a) What term is given to the tongue abnormality?
(b) What abnormality is shown in the stool concentrate?
(c) What is the underlying diagnosis?

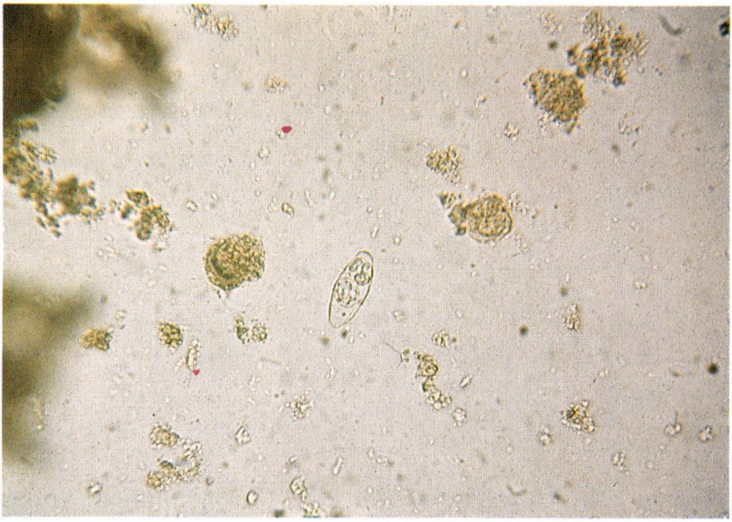

129

130

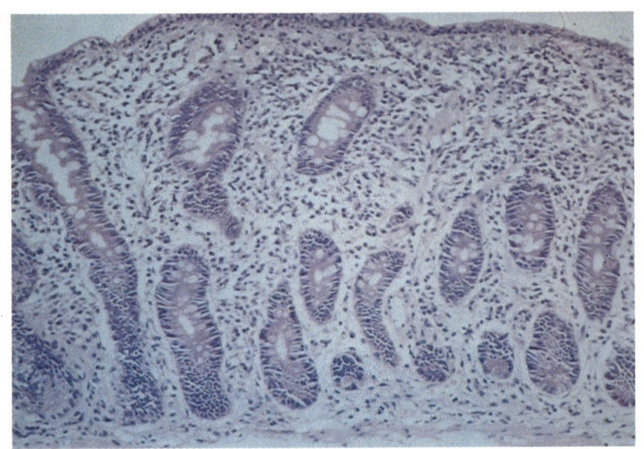

130 This photomicrograph is from a jejunal biopsy taken from a 57-year-old woman with diarrhoea.
(a) What is the most significant feature on the biopsy?
(b) What is the most likely diagnosis?
(c) How is this diagnosis confirmed?

131

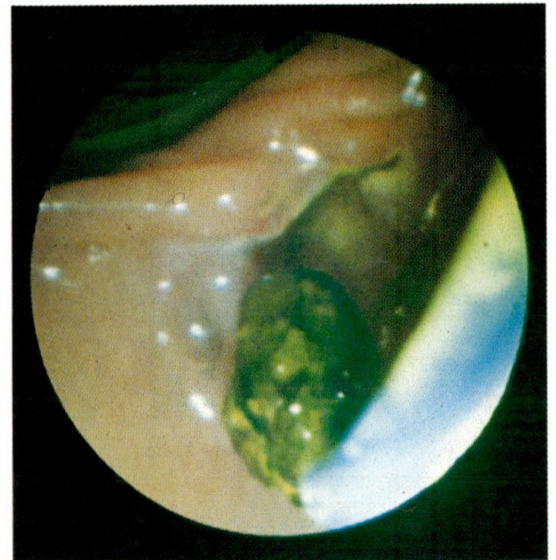

131 This photograph was taken during ERCP in a 38-year-old woman with acute pancreatitis.
(a) What procedures have been performed?
(b) What are the three most important potential complications of these procedures?
(c) In what circumstances might ERCP be indicated early in the course of acute pancreatitis?

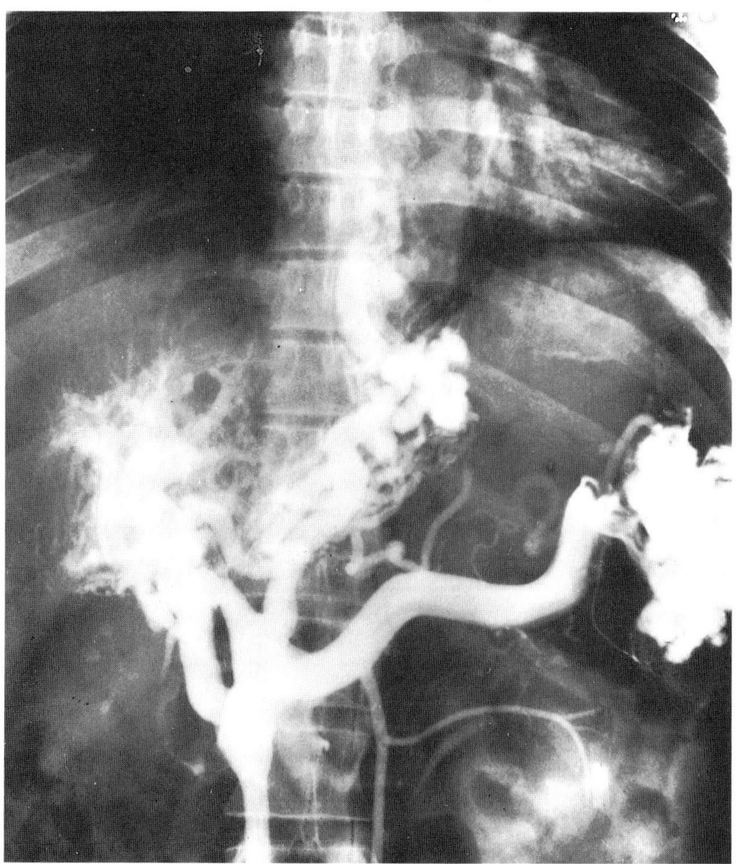

132 A 38-year-old man with a history of two recent upper gastrointestinal bleeds underwent radiological evaluation. He was a heavy smoker, but gave no history of alcohol excess. His only past medical history was resection of a bleeding Meckel's diverticulum 20 years previously.

(a) What investigation is being performed?

(b) What is the most likely source of the recent bleeding?

(c) What underlying disease is probably responsible for the appearances seen here?

133

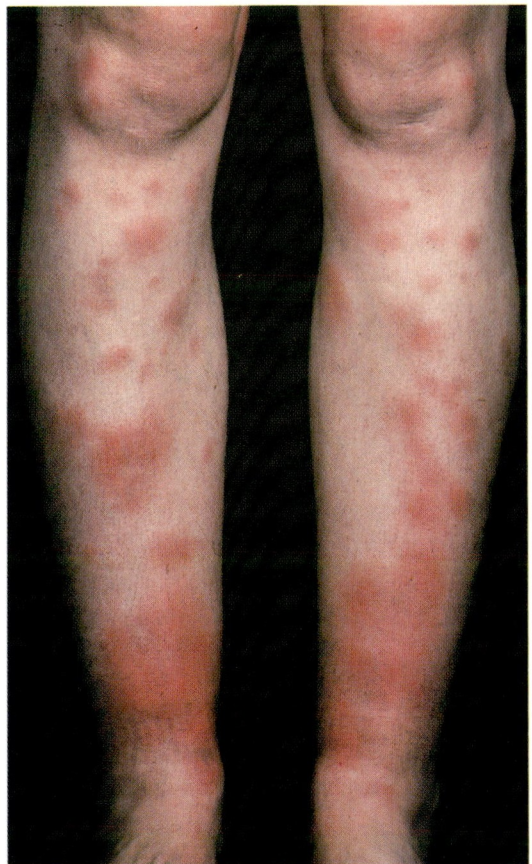

133 A 26-year-old woman with a two-month history of diarrhoea presented with this eruption on the legs. She had recently been taking antibiotics for a sore throat. She smoked heavily and was a regular user of the oral contraceptive pill. She worked in a stocking factory.

(a) What is this eruption?

(b) Give five possible predisposing factors in this patient.

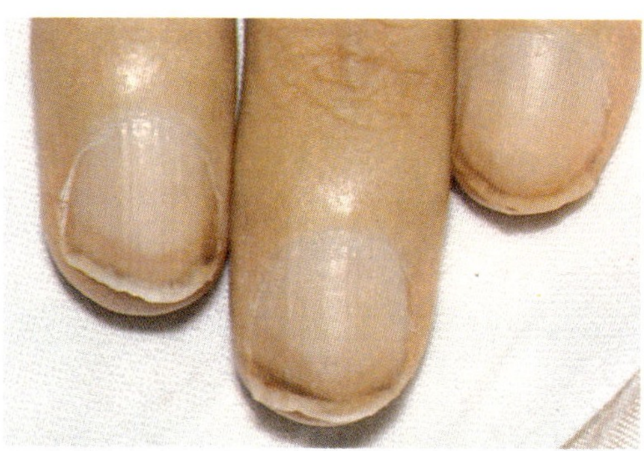

134

134 This is from a 58-year-old man with a history of recent ankle swelling.
(a) What abnormality is shown?
(b) What metabolic abnormality is thought to be responsible for this appearance?
(c) Give two possible underlying diseases.

135 A 19-year-old student in biochemistry was referred with a painful swelling in his mouth. He had lost 5 kg in weight. Past medical history included arthritis in the right knee and perianal abscess.
(a) What name is given to the buccal abnormality?
(b) What is the probable underlying diagnosis?

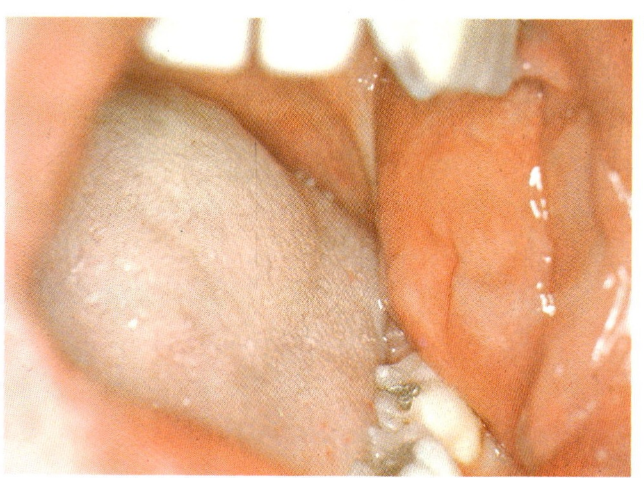

135

136

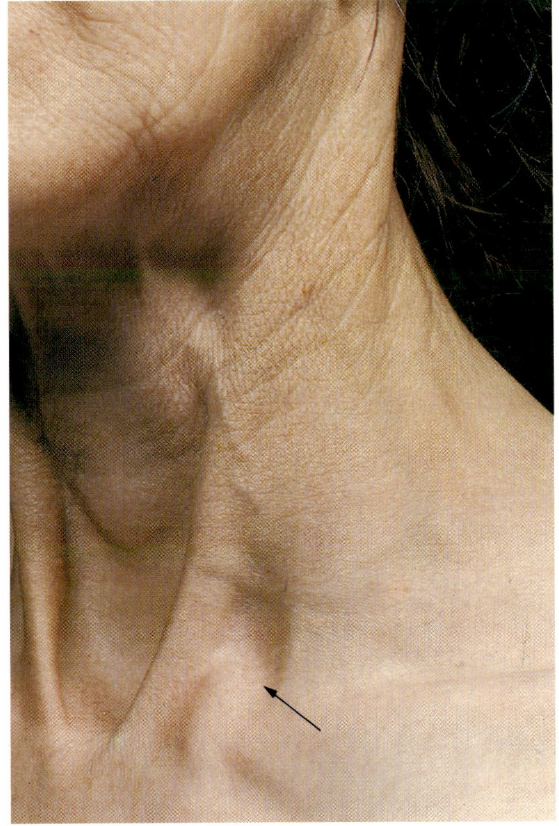

136 A 60-year-old woman complained of having lost 8 kg in weight over three months. She was found to have a haemoglobin concentration of 8g/dl and a hypochromic, microcytic blood film.

(a) What abnormality is shown?

(b) What is the probable underlying diagnosis?

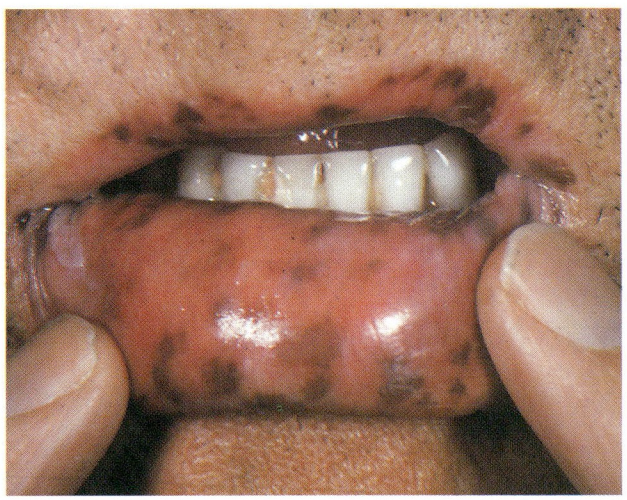

137

137 A 24-year-old man was referred with recurrent anaemia.
(a) What is the diagnosis?
(b) What is the cause of the recurrent anaemia?
(c) Give two other complications of this disorder.

138

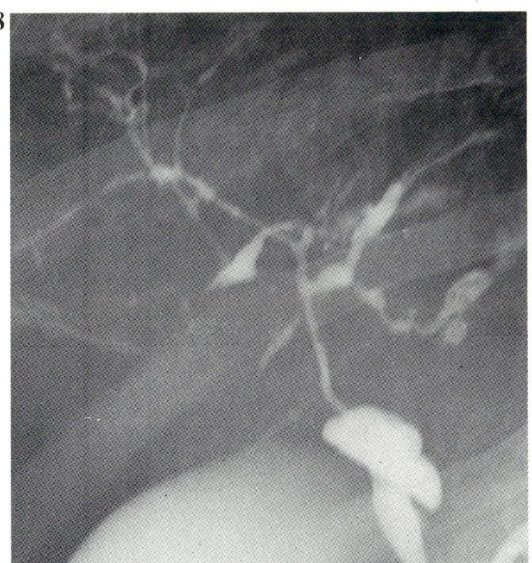

138 A 42-year-old man was referred with painless progressive jaundice and recurrent fever.
(a) What investigation has been performed?
(b) Describe the abnormalities on this X-ray.
(c) What is the diagnosis?
(d) Which associated gastrointestinal disease may also be present in this man?

139

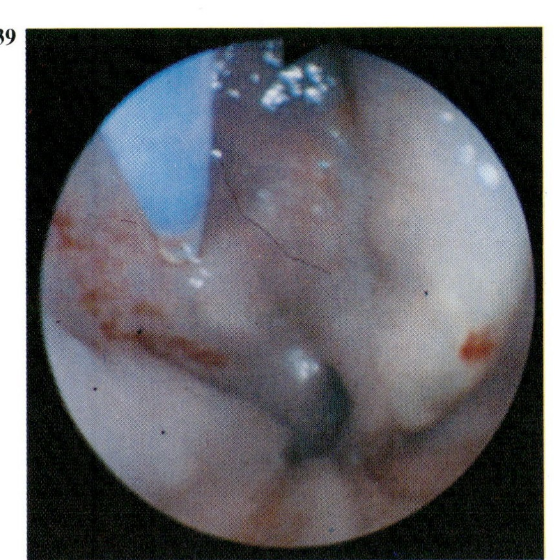

139 A 69-year-old woman was endoscoped following a recent haematemesis.
(a) What procedure is being performed?
(b) What are the two commonest complications of this procedure?

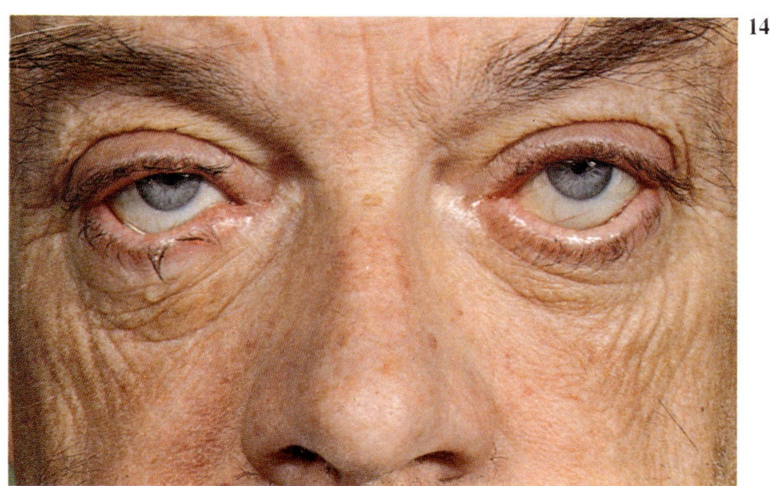

140

140, 141 A 65-year-old man was referred with a two-year history of lacrimation and profuse watery diarrhoea. He had not lost weight. His liver edge was palpable 15 cm below the right costal margin and felt hard and irregular. His chest X-ray is illustrated in **141**.

(a) What is the probable diagnosis?

(b) Give three possible approaches to relieving his symptoms.

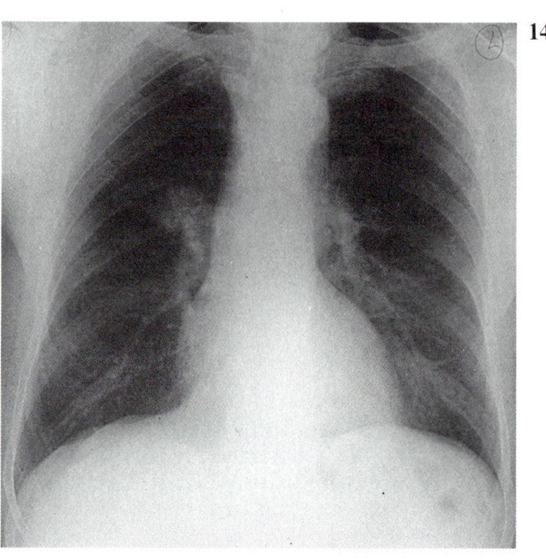

141

142

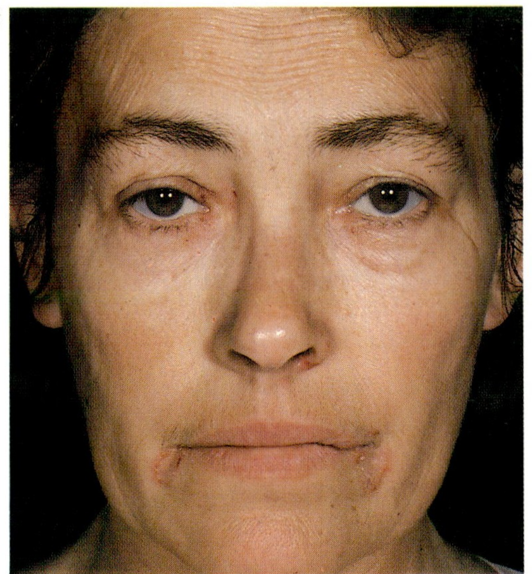

143

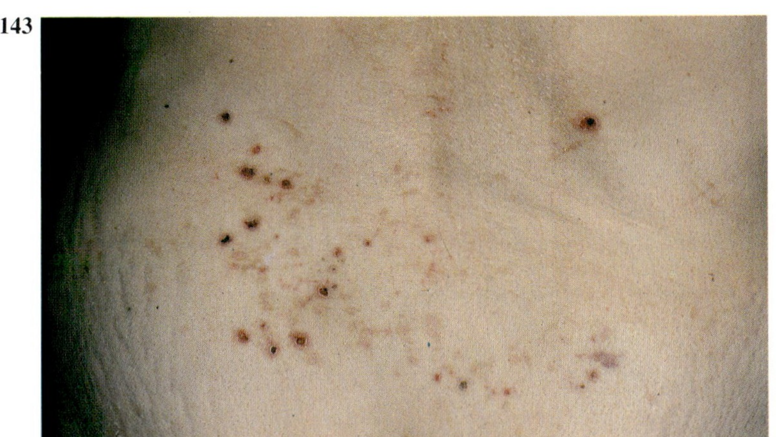

142, 143 A 48-year-old woman complained of tiredness, weight loss, itching and increased stool frequency.

(a) What two abnormal features are evident from **142**?
(b) What do these two features indicate?
(c) What is the skin eruption in **143**?
(d) What is the underlying diagnosis?

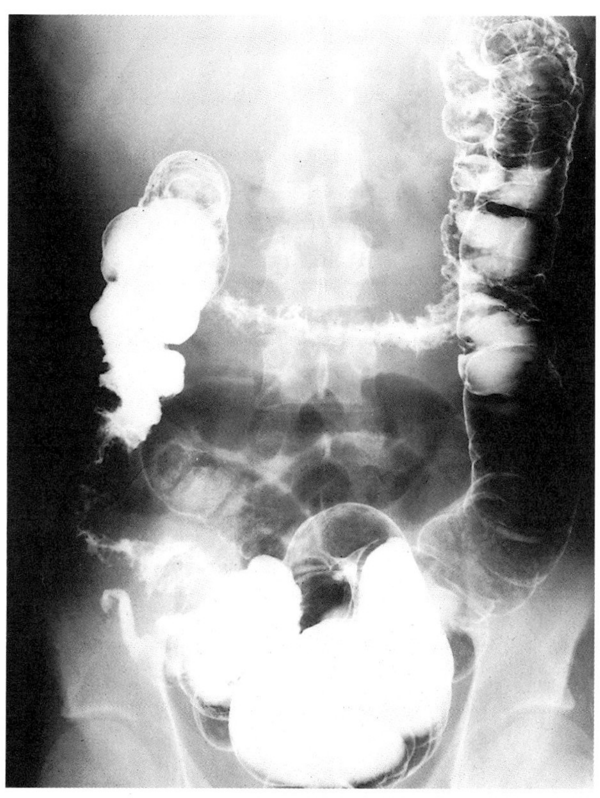

144

144 This barium enema was performed in a 22-year-old man with a three-month history of diarrhoea and colicky central abdominal pain.
(a) What abnormalities are shown?
(b) What is the probable diagnosis?

145

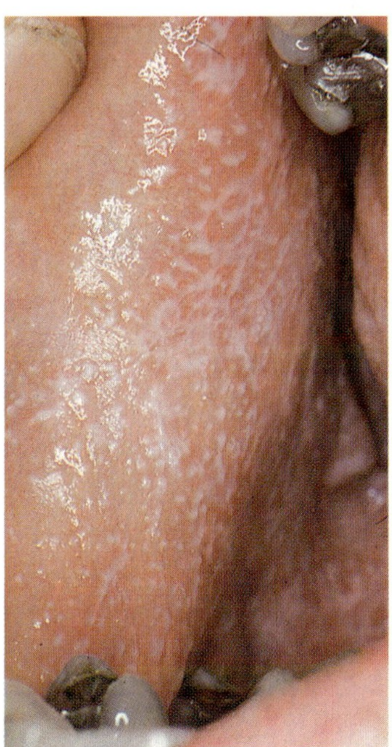

145 A 56-year-old woman was referred for investigation of dysphagia. On examination there was a papular purplish eruption over the wrists and forearms. The appearance of the buccal mucosa is illustrated.

(a) What is the diagnosis?

(b) What oesophageal manifestations of this disorder are recognised?

(c) What treatment should be considered?

146 A young woman gave a two-week history of fever and sore throat. She was found to have cervical lymphadenopathy and an enlarged liver on examination. Ten days later, she presented with this diffuse maculo-papular eruption.

(a) What is the most likely diagnosis?

(b) What was the likely precipitant of the eruption?

146

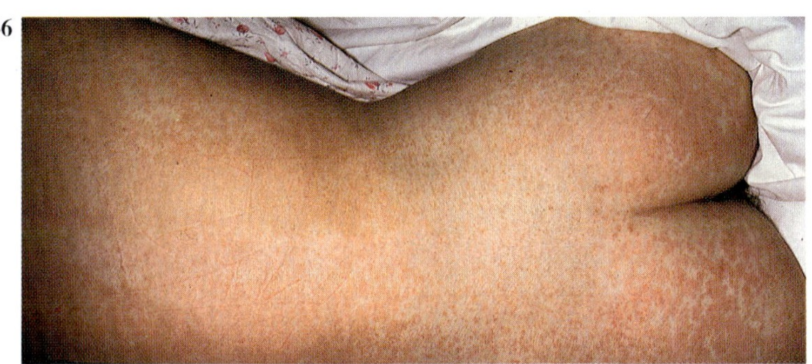

147 A 35-year-old woman presented with haematemesis and melaena. Her elbow flexures had an unusual appearance.
(a) What is the diagnosis?
(b) Where else, apart from the skin, would you look for signs of this disorder?
(c) Why does gastrointestinal haemorrhage develop in this condition?

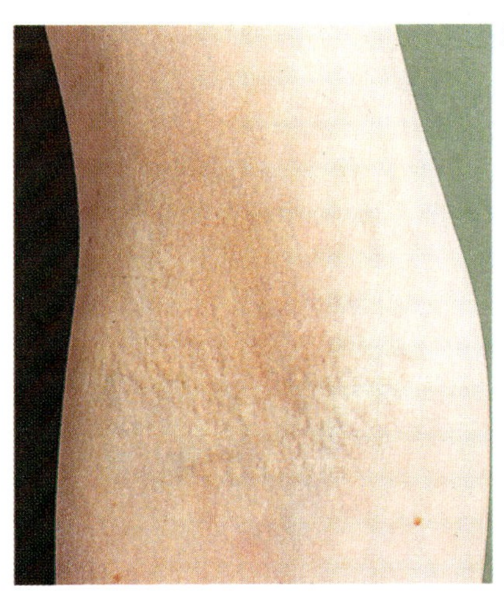
147

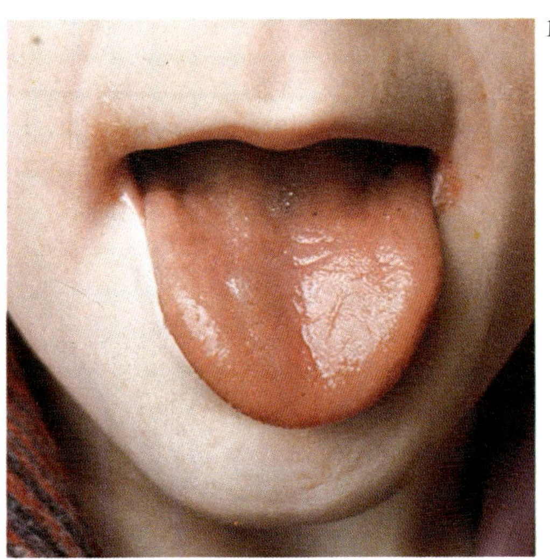
148

148 An 18-year-old woman was referred for investigation of chronic lethargy and diarrhoea.
(a) What two abnormalities are apparent in this photograph?
(b) What is the likely explanation for lethargy?
(c) Apart from routine physical examination, which three clinical procedures might help to elicit the cause of her symptoms?

149

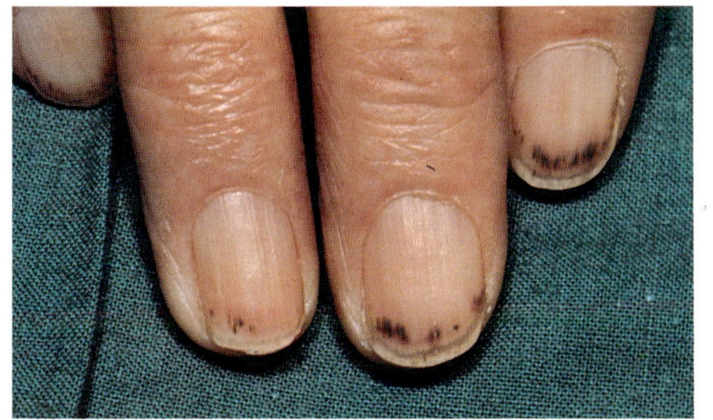

149 A 64-year-old woman presented with abdominal pain, followed by the passage of a dark red stool per rectum. Although her spleen was slightly enlarged, the appearance of her fingernails was the most striking feature on examination.
(a) What abnormality is shown?
(b) What diagnosis do you suspect?
(c) How have the abdominal symptoms arisen?

150 (a) What is this piece of equipment used for?
(b) What is the main complication associated with its use?

150

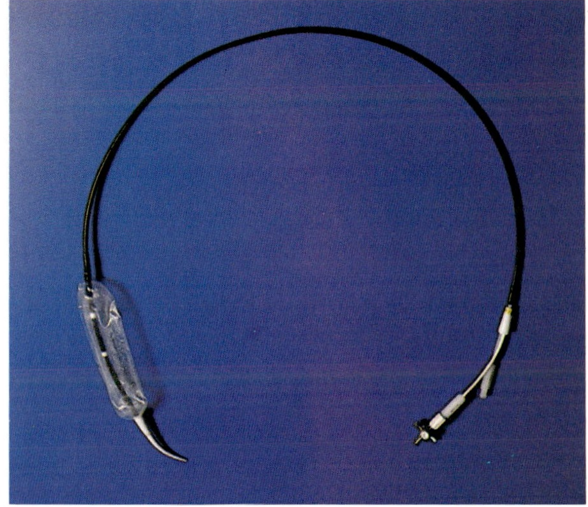

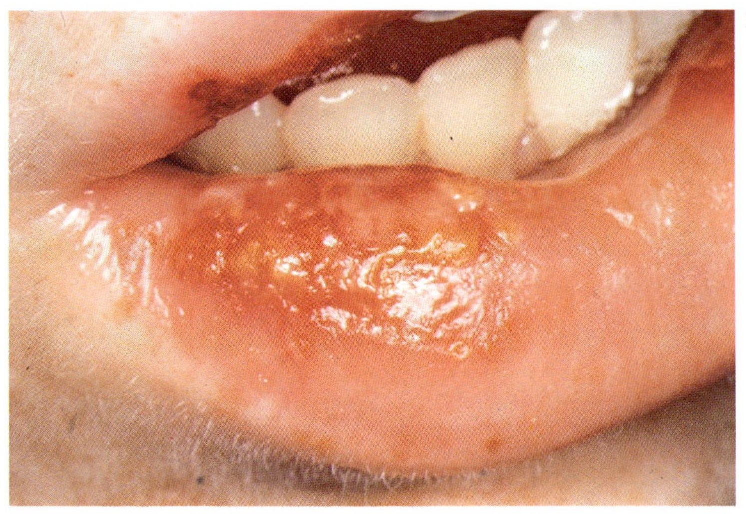
151

151, 152 These are the mouth and hands of a 37-year-old woman with coeliac disease and intestinal lymphoma who had been receiving intravenous feeding for six weeks.
(a) What is the cause of the abnormalities shown here?
(b) How is this diagnosis confirmed?

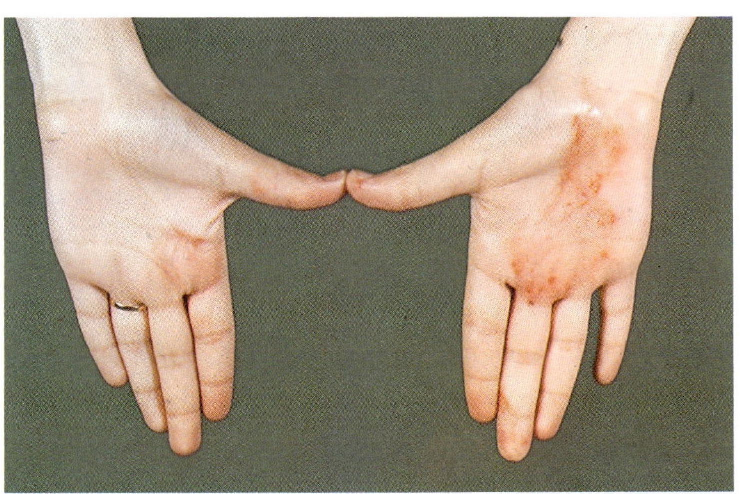
152

153

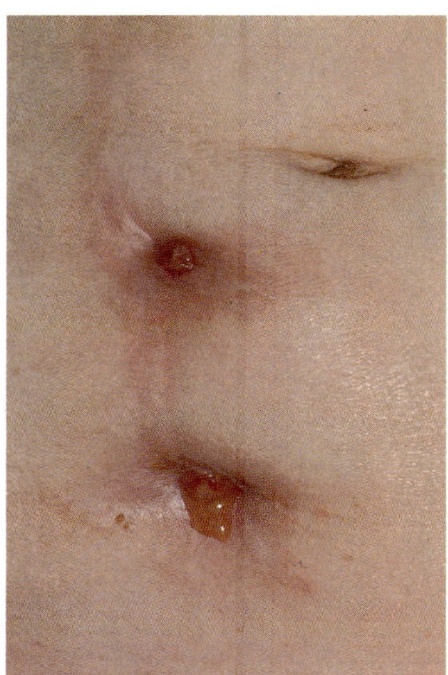

153 A 46-year-old woman had previously undergone a small bowel resection for Crohn's disease.
(a) What complication has developed?
(b) How may this be confirmed?

154

154 This 26-year-old man was receiving treatment for coeliac disease and dermatitis herpetiformis. He noted that his tongue and extremities had recently become darker. Arterial blood gas concentrations were normal.
(a) What has caused the change in colour?
(b) What might have precipitated this phenomenon?

155 A 17-year-old man was referred for dietary assessment. Since he left home one year previously, he had mainly existed on a diet of peanut-butter sandwiches.
(a) What is the cause of the skin changes?
(b) Where else would you look for confirmation of this disorder?
(c) How is this diagnosis confirmed biochemically?

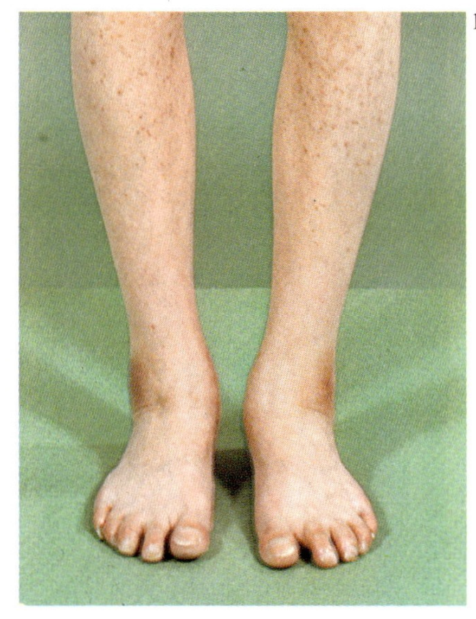

155

156 (a) What investigation is being performed?
(b) What are the two main advantages of this investigation over more traditional X-ray imaging?

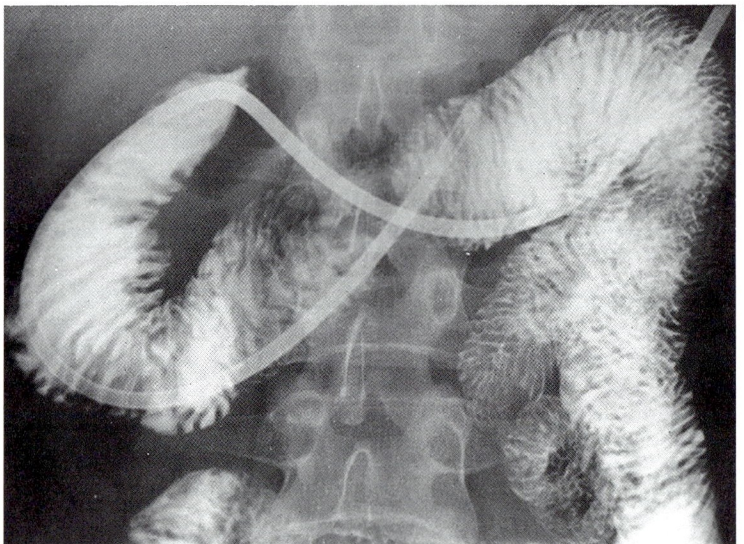

156

157

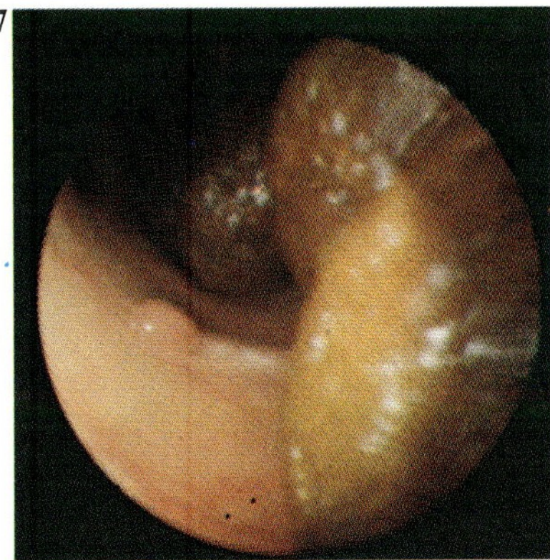

157 A 68-year-old man reported the recent onset of constipation and underwent out-patient flexible sigmoidoscopy.
(a) What abnormality is shown?
(b) What action should be taken by the sigmoidoscopist?

158

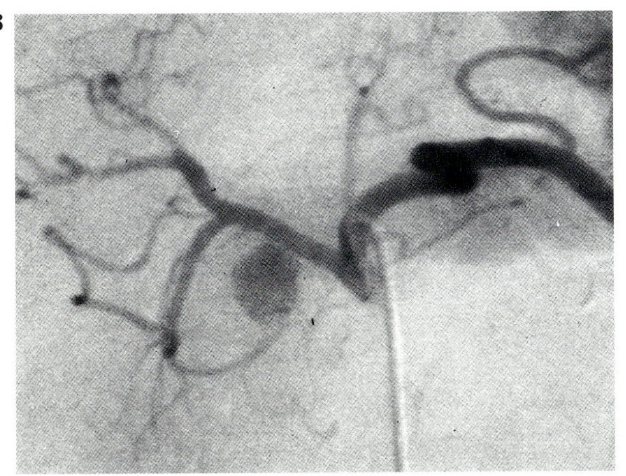

158 A 46-year-old man was arrested, apparently drunk and disorderly. His wife, accompanying him, stated that he had not been drinking, but that he had recently been experiencing episodes of sweating and had developed an increased appetite. The patient become unconscious in the police cell and was transferred to hospital for investigation.
(a) What investigation is being performed?
(b) What is the diagnosis?

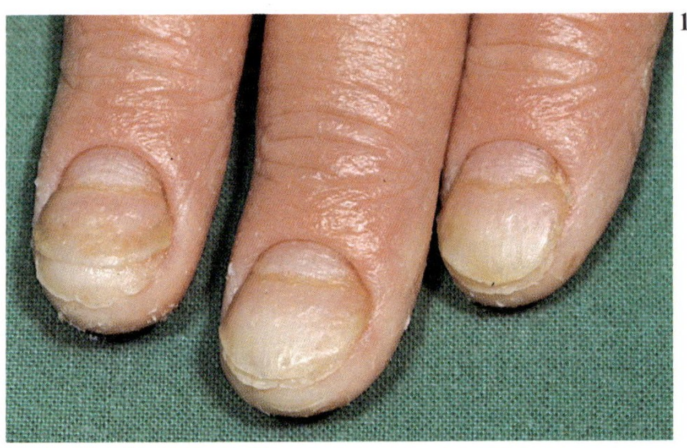
159

159 A 46-year-old man was transferred from the dermatology ward because he had recently developed ascites.
(a) What has caused these nail changes?
(b) Which preventable complication may have caused his ascites?

160 A 16-year-old male was referred for investigation of short stature, lack of pubertal development and recent proximal muscle weakness. He was found to be anaemic, and three stool samples were positive for occult blood.
(a) Which gastroenterological disorder should be considered?
(b) Give five relevant investigations.

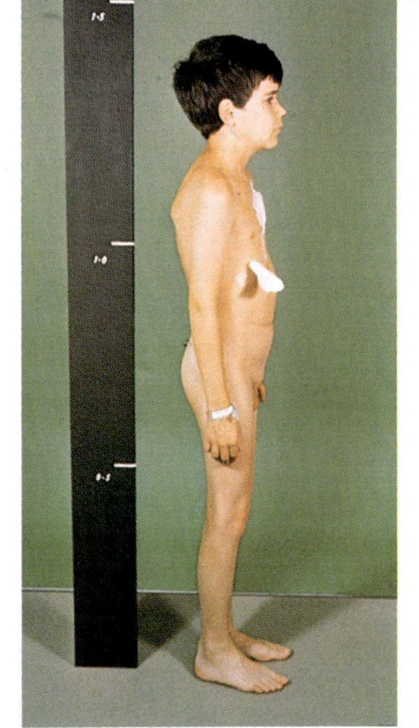
160

161

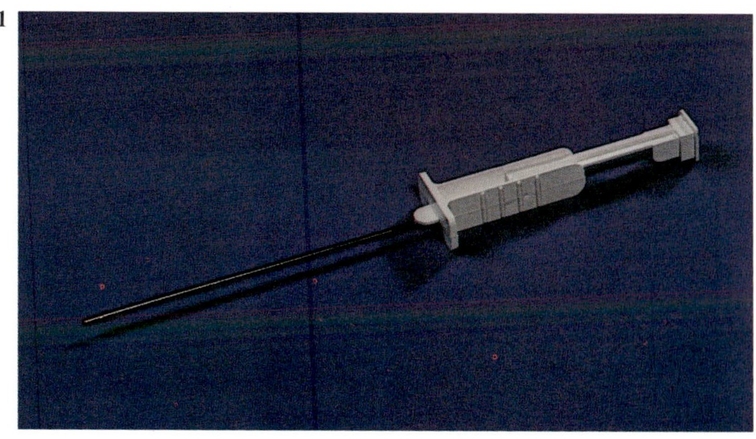

161 (a) What is this device?
(b) Give its two most common uses in gastroenterological practice.

162

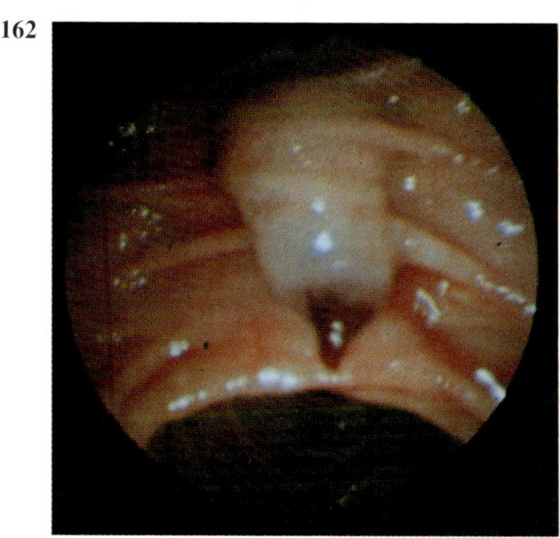

163

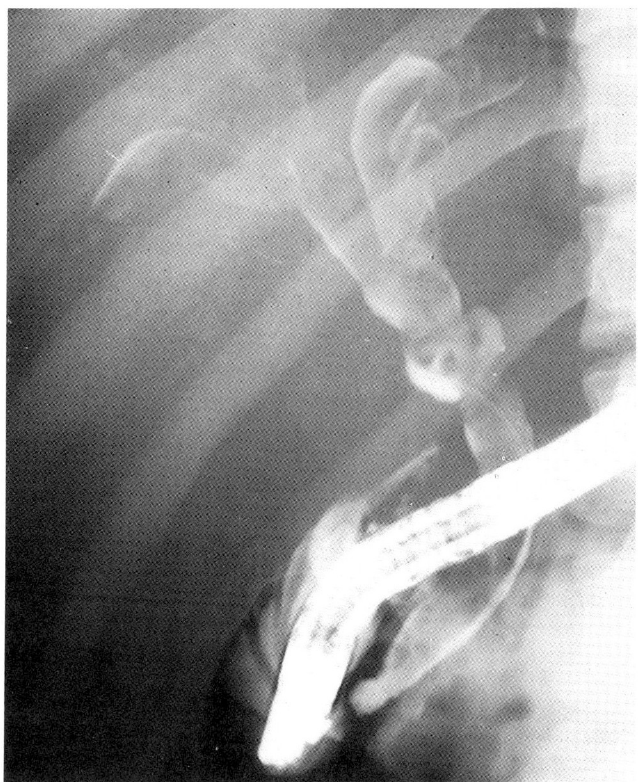

162, 163 A 36-year-old man was admitted for investigation of abnormal liver function tests. Upper abdominal ultrasound was normal. It was decided to perform percutaneous liver biopsy, followed by endoscopic retrograde cholangiography. The appearance of the ampulla of Vater prior to cholangiography is shown in **162**, and **163** demonstrates the cholangiographic appearances.

(a) What phenomenon has been demonstrated?

(b) What had led to the development of this phenomenon?

164

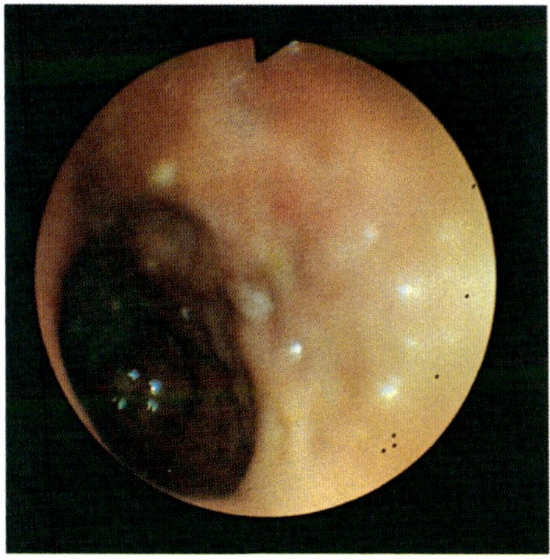

164, 165 A colonoscopic view from a 32-year-old man with a four-week history of diarrhoea and rectal bleeding. He had returned from Ethiopia three months previously, but stool cultures were negative. Part of a colonoscopic biopsy specimen is illustrated in **165**.
(a) What is the diagnosis?
(b) What treatment would you advise?

165

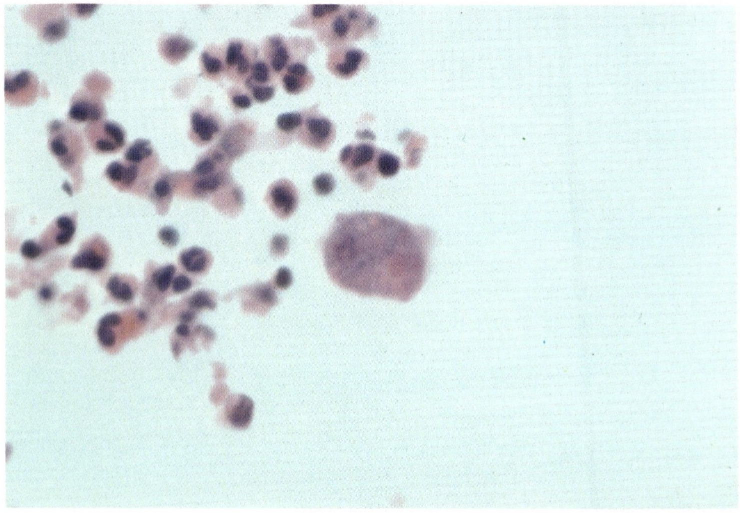

166 A 42-year-old man complained of perianal pain on defaecation and occasional rectal bleeding.
(a) What abnormality is shown on inspection of the anus?
(b) What is the most likely predisposing factor?

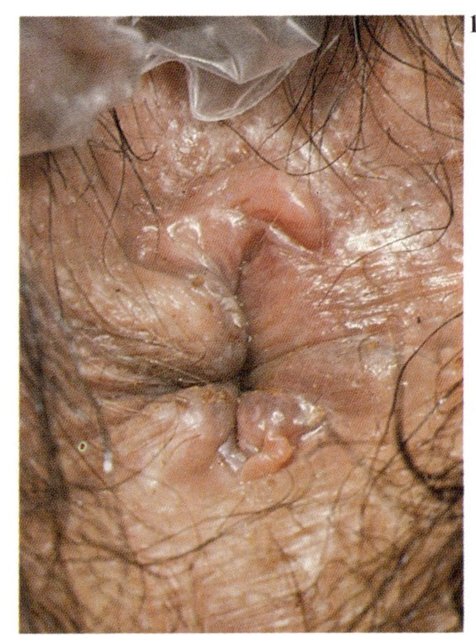
166

167 A two-month-old infant with intermittent vomiting of feed underwent infusion of barium via a nasogastric tube. An oblique radiograph was obtained.
(a) What abnormality is shown?
(b) Give two possible associated congenital disorders.

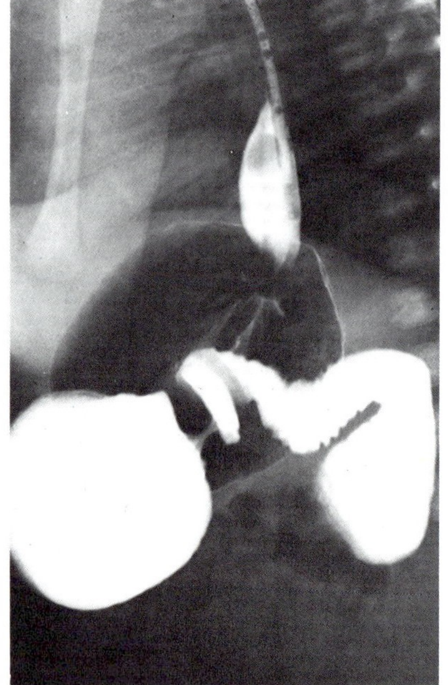
167

168 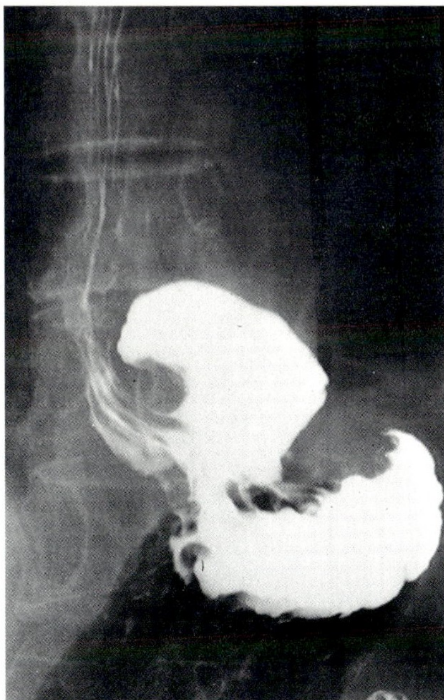

168 A 64-year-old woman with recurrent epigastric pain underwent barium meal examination.
(a) What abnormality is identified?
(b) What treatment should be considered?

169 This patient gave a two-day history of diarrhoea and rectal bleeding. The only abnormal finding on sigmoidoscopy was the presence of dark red blood in the rectal lumen.
(a) What operation has previously been performed?
(b) What disease was likely to have caused the rectal bleeding?

169 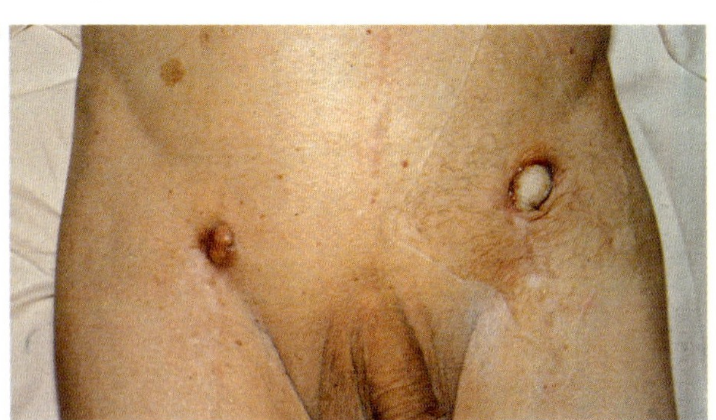

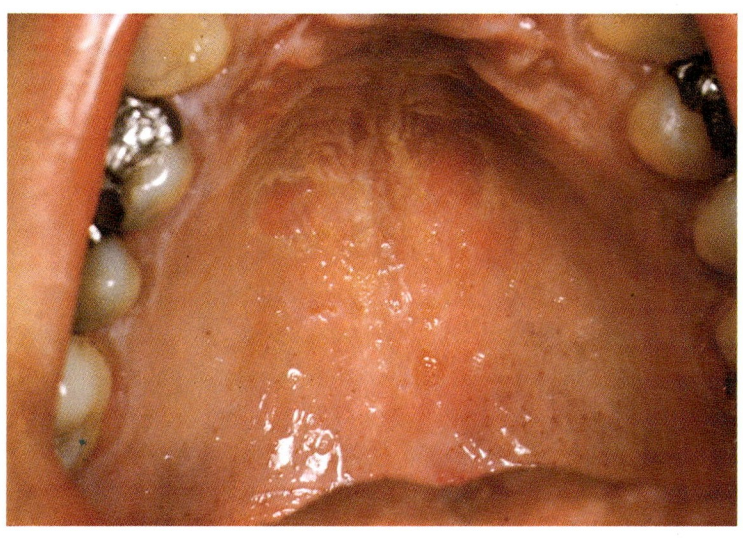

170

170 A 22-year-old man developed a maculopapular rash, generalised lymphadenopathy and mild fever. Liver function tests showed marked elevation of plasma alkaline phosphatase activity. Inspection of the hard palate revealed ulceration, which had been painless.
(a) What is the diagnosis?
(b) How is this confirmed?

171 This view was obtained during endoscopic inspection of the lower oesophagus in a patient with a recent small haematemesis.
(a) What abnormality is shown?
(b) Give two possible predisposing factors.

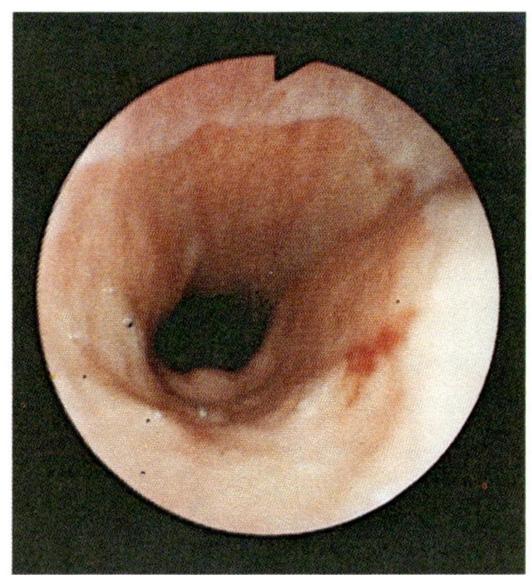

171

172

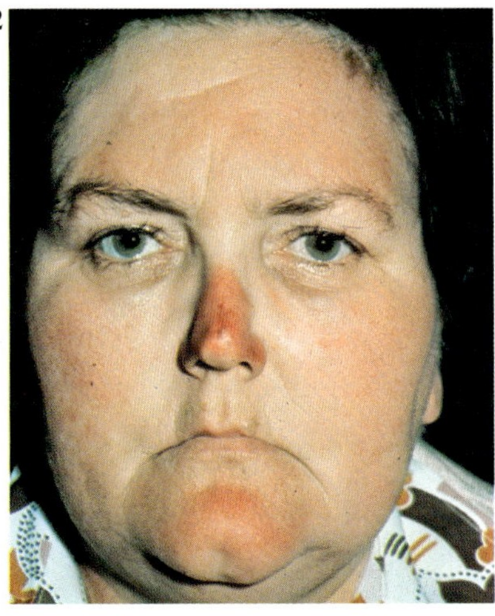

172 A 52-year-old woman presented with recurring colicky abdominal pain associated with intermittent redness and swelling of the nose and lips. Her mother had suffered similarly.
(a) What is this rare hereditary disorder?
(b) What confirmatory investigation may be helpful?

173 A 32-year-old man with ankylosing spondylitis developed intermittent epigastric discomfort, especially at night.
(a) What abnormality is shown on this barium meal?
(b) What is the most likely predisposing factor?
(c) How is the diagnosis confirmed?

173

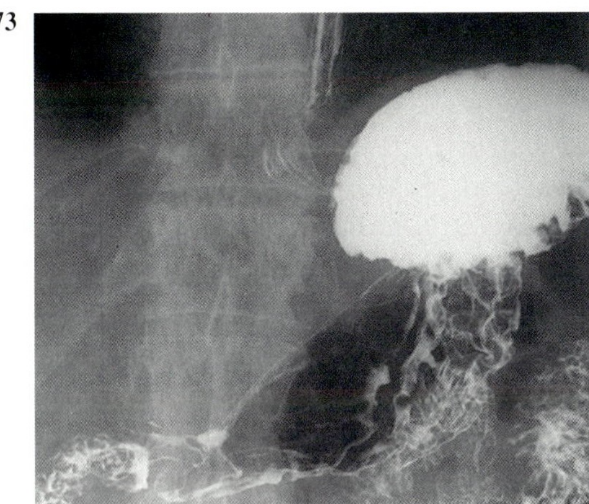

174 A 68-year-old woman presented with haematemesis. She did not consume alcohol and had previously been well.
(a) Which three clinical features are noteworthy from her facial appearance?
(b) What is the most likely diagnosis?
(c) What is the likely cause of haematemesis?

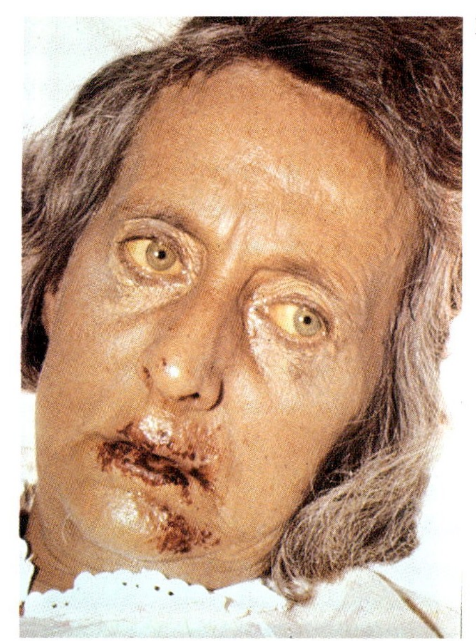
174

175 A 56-year-old divorced night-club owner developed painful breast enlargement. He had been treated for ascites and oedema during the preceding two years.
(a) What is the probable underlying diagnosis?
(b) Which drug may have aggravated his breast tenderness?

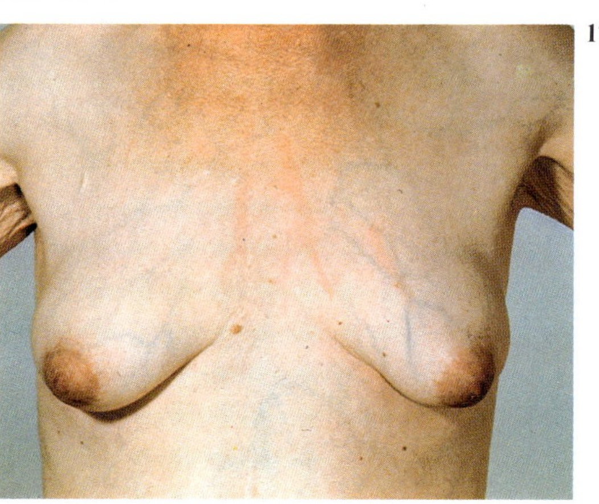
175

176

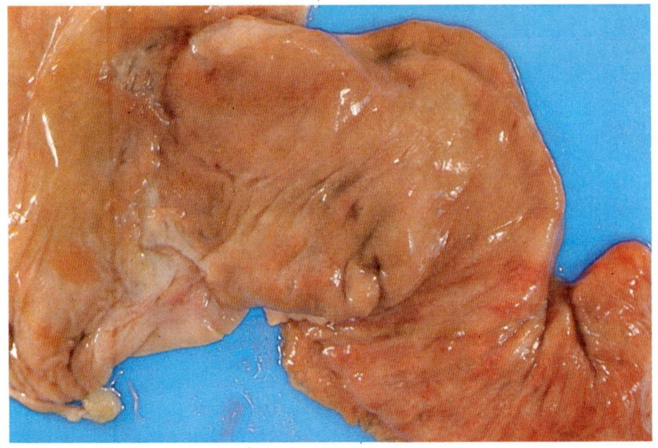

176 This specimen of terminal ileum and caecum was resected from a 74-year-old woman with a history of iron-deficiency anaemia and recent passage of altered blood per rectum. There are two ulcers in the terminal ileum, the largest of which is involving the ileocaecal valve.
(a) Which two classes of drug have been linked to small intestinal ulceration and haemorrhage?
(b) Give two other possible complications of small intestinal ulcers.

177

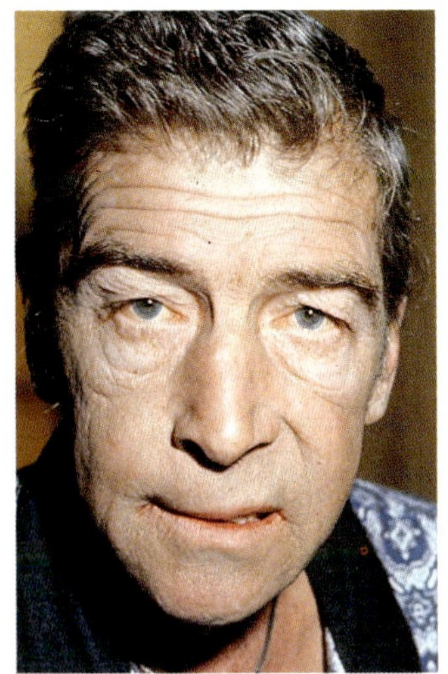

177 This 56-year-old man developed diabetes mellitus. There was no history of alcohol excess. Examination of the abdomen revealed an enlarged liver, which was smooth and non-tender.
(a) What is the diagnosis?
(b) What is the treatment?
(c) Which important late complication is not prevented by this treatment?

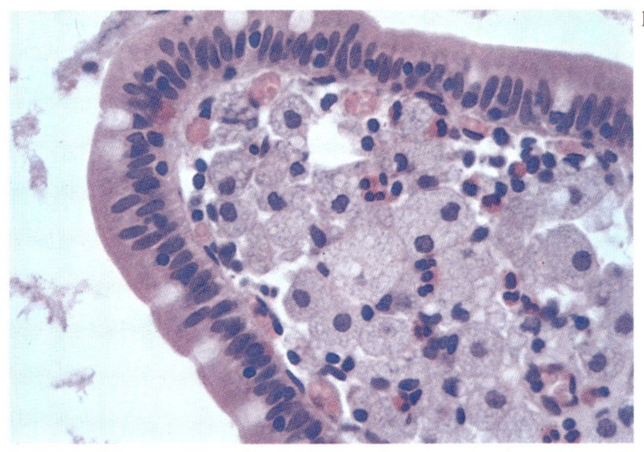 178

178 This photomicrograph of a jejunal villus was taken from a man with a rare disease characterised by malabsorption, pigmentation, arthritis and fever.
(a) What is the diagnosis?
(b) How is this disorder treated?

179 A 38-year-old woman had become increasingly jaundiced over two months. There was no history of foreign traval or contacts with hepatitis. She did not drink alcohol and had been on no medications. Virus serology was negative. Biochemical investigations confirmed jaundice, with marked elevations of serum transaminase activities.
(a) List four further relevant non-invasive investigations.
(b) Which rare hereditary disorder must be excluded?

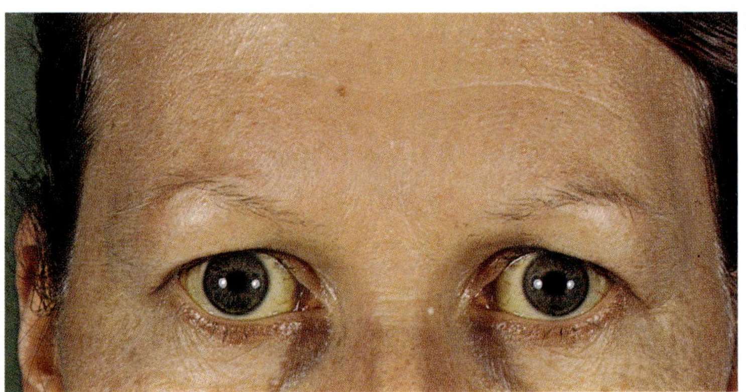 179

180

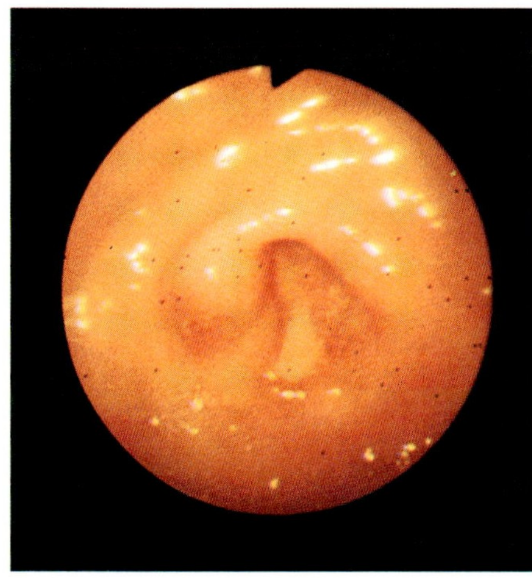

180 This endoscopic photograph was obtained from a 36-year-old man with a previously diagnosed pre-pyloric ulcer which had failed to heal after three months of treatment with high-dose anti-secretory drug therapy.
(a) Give three possible reasons why the ulcer has failed to heal.
(b) Give two relevant further investigations.

181 This young woman developed recurrent severe ulceration of the mouth and tongue in association with a painful red eye.
(a) What is the diagnosis?
(b) Which three other parts of the body are commonly affected in this disease?

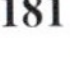

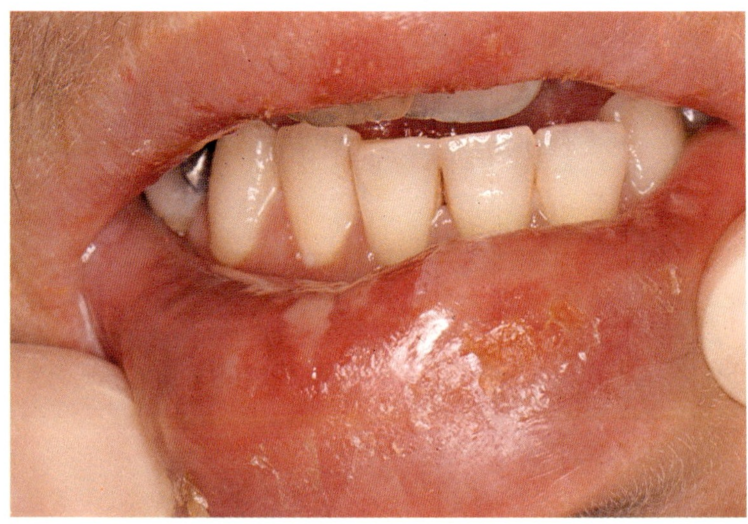

182, 183 A 62-year-old woman presented to a dental hospital with a history of repeated tongue-biting. She had also suffered back pain and occasional pale stools during the last six months. Haemoglobin was reduced at 9g/dl. Blood film showed rouleaux formation. Erythrocyte sedimentation rate was 150 mm in the first hour. The photomicrograph **183** is of a rectal biopsy specimen stained to represent the characteristic features of an uncommon systemic disease.

(a) What features are demonstrated on inspection of her tongue?

(b) What condition can be diagnosed from the rectal biopsy?

(c) What is the underlying diagnosis?

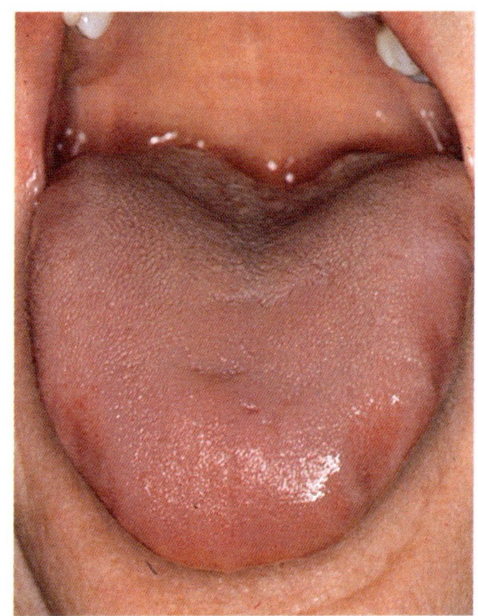

182

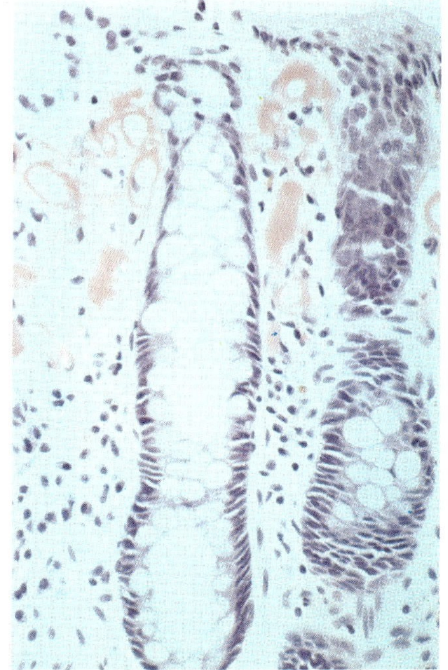

183

Answers

94, 95 (a) Graft-versus-host disease.
(b) Rectal biopsy.
(c) Infective causes should be excluded by microscopy and the culture of stools and testing them for *Clostridium difficile* toxin.

96 (a) Multiple cysts within the liver.
(b) Hydatid disease.
(c) Indirect haemagglutination and complement fixation tests are available, but fail to detect antibody in the serum in 15% of cases.

97 (a) Bruising around venepuncture sites might be due to a prolonged prothrombin time due to liver dysfunction and/or a low platelet count due to hypersplenism.
(b) Reduced total lung capacity due to ascites and pleural fluid; functional arterio-venous shunting due to end-stage liver disease; aspiration pneumonia; alpha$_1$-antitrypsin deficiency, leading to emphysema.

98 (a) Pneumatosis cystoides intestinalis.
(b) Chronic bronchitis and emphysema.
(c) Continuous high-flow oxygen.

99 (a) Localised dilatation of the main pancreatic duct and its side branches in the tail of the pancreas.
(b) Chronic pancreatitis.

100 (a) Perianal abscess.
(b) Incision and drainage under general anaesthesia.

101 (a) Carcinoma of the stomach.
(b) Endoscopic biopsy.
(c) Atrophic gastritis, gastric adenomatous polyps, previous gastric surgery, including vagotomy and drainage.

102 (a) Previous surgery (choledochoduodenostomy or choledochojejunostomy).
(b) Ascending cholangitis.
(c) Retrograde flow of small bowel contents through the anastomosis; a sump syndrome with stasis in the common bile duct distal to the anastomosis.

103 (a) Primary hepatocellular carcinoma associated with longstanding chronic carriage of the hepatitis B virus. He had become an asymptomatic hepatitis B carrier following tattoo-marking in the Far East.
(b) Hepatitis B surface antigen, alpha-fetoprotein level, imaging procedure (ultrasound or computerised tomography).

104 (a) Niche of barium in the first part of the duodenum with folds radiating towards it.
(b) Duodenal ulcer.

105 (a) Primary biliary cirrhosis.
(b) Liver function tests, serum anti-mitochondrial antibodies, liver biopsy.

106 (a) Ulcerative colitis.
(b) Toxic dilatation of the colon.
(c) Sigmoidoscopy, rectal biopsy, stool assay for *Clostridium difficile* toxin.

107 (a) Degos' disease (malignant atrophic papulosis).
(b) Intestinal perforation.

108 (a) Pharyngeal pouch.
(b) Aspiration pneumonia.
(c) No. Endoscopy has little or nothing to add and is potentially hazardous—inadvertent intubation of the diverticulum could lead to perforation.
(d) Surgical excision of the pouch.

109 (a) Oral candidiasis.
(b) Infection with the human immunodeficiency virus, leading to the acquired immune deficiency syndrome (AIDS).
(c) Poor oral hygiene, broad spectrum antibiotics, immunosuppression, diabetes mellitus.

110 (a) Aphthoid ulceration.
(b) Crohn's disease.
(c) Seronegative arthritis associated with inflammatory bowel disease.

111 (a) Carcinoma of the head of the pancreas.
(b) Either endoscopic endoprosthesis insertion or surgical by-pass.

112 (a) Anal carcinoma.
(b) Human papillomavirus 16.
(c) Initial radiotherapy, perhaps followed by surgery.

113, 114 (a) Villous adenoma.
(b) Hypokalaemia.

115 (a) Small intestinal obstruction.
(b) Inguinal or femoral hernia, adhesions from previous surgery.

116 (a) Enterocolic fistula.
(b) Carcinoma of the colon.
(c) Transit of small bowel contents through the fistula and into the large bowel, together with bacterial overgrowth in the small intestine.

117 (a) Grey Turner's sign.
(b) Acute pancreatitis.
(c) Retroperitoneal haemorrhage.

118 (a) Bronchial carcinoma. Oesophageal carcinoma is a less likely possibility.
(b) Tracheo-oesophageal fistula.
(c) Endoscopic placement of an oesophageal tube (see **5**).

119 (a) T-tube cholangiography.
(b) Ascaris lumbricoides worm in the common bile duct.
(c) Systemic antihelminthic drugs; infusion of piperazine citrate via the T-tube; retrieval of the offending worm, either via the T-tube or endoscopically after papillotomy.

120 (a) Leiomyoma of the stomach.
(b) Sarcomatous change.
(c) Surgical wedge excision.

121 (a) Vasculitic lesions on the right great toe.
(b) Fingers, nail beds, optic fundi.
(c) Infective endocarditis; polyarteritis nodosa in association with chronic hepatitis B.

122 (a) Displacement of the upper and lower sections of the second part of the duodenum by an extrinsic mass lying medially. This is the so-called reverse-3 appearance.
(b) Pancreatic carcinoma.

123 (a) Replacement of the lower oesophageal epithelium by gastric columnar epithelium. The junction between the two types of mucosa is irregular.
(b) Barrett's oesophagus.
(c) Malignant change, oesophageal ulcer, benign oesophageal stricture.

124 (a) Amoebic liver abscess.
(b) Amoebic serology, microscopy of fresh stool specimen.
(c) Metronidazole.

125 (a) Peristomal varices.
(b) Portal hypertension due to primary sclerosing cholangitis.

126 (a) Carcinoma of the sigmoid colon.
(b) Colonoscopy can be used to obtain biopsies for histological confirmation pre-operatively and, more importantly in this case, to follow the patient post-operatively for detection (and possible treatment) of synchronous or metachronous colonic neoplasia.

127 (a) Multiple small post-inflammatory polyps (pseudopolyps).
(b) Multiple pseudopolyps are commonly found in colitis patients and do not in themselves affect management.
(c) Inactive; the vascular pattern is well preserved.

128, 129 (a) Hairy leucoplakia.
(b) Oocyst of *Isospora belli* in the centre of the field.
(c) Acquired immune deficiency syndrome (AIDS).

130 (a) Subtotal villous atrophy.
(b) Coeliac disease (gluten-sensitive enteropathy).
(c) The patient is commenced on a gluten-free diet, and a follow-up biopsy is done six months later to confirm that the histological appearance is returning to normal.

131 (a) Endoscopic sphincterotomy and removal of a gallstone.
(b) Haemorrhage or perforation after sphincterotomy; risk of introducing infection into bile duct or pancreas.
(c) Severe pancreatitis thought to be due to gallstones.

132 (a) Splenoportography.
(b) Oesophageal varices.
(c) Chronic liver disease resulting from previous blood transfusion.

133 (a) Erythema nodosum.
(b) Ulcerative colitis, Crohn's disease, streptococcal infection, Epstein–Barr virus infection, sulphonamide therapy, oral contraceptive usage.

134 (a) Leuconychia (white nails).
(b) Hypoalbuminaemia.
(c) Cirrhosis, nephrotic syndrome.

135 (a) Orofacial granulomatosis.
(b) Crohn's disease.

136 (a) Left supraclavicular lymphadenopathy.
(b) Carcinoma of lower oesophagus or stomach.

137 (a) Peutz–Jeghers syndrome.
(b) Multiple gastrointestinal polyps.
(c) Intussusception of small bowel polyps, increased cancer risk (gastrointestinal and extraintestinal neoplasms).

138 (a) Endoscopic retrograde cholangio-pancreatography (ERCP).
(b) Multiple strictures affecting the intrahepatic bile ducts and the common hepatic duct. Localised dilatations of the intrahepatic ducts are also demonstrated.
(c) Primary sclerosing cholangitis.
(d) Ulcerative colitis.

139 (a) Endoscopic sclerotherapy of oesophageal varices.
(b) Sclerosis ulceration, oesophageal stricture.

140, 141 (a) Bronchial carcinoid tumour with liver metastases, leading to the carcinoid syndrome.
(b) Serotonin antagonists, subcutaneous octreotide and hepatic artery embolisation. Chemotherapy with interferon and/or 5-fluorouracil may be helpful.

142, 143 (a) Blue sclerae, angular cheilitis.
(b) Iron deficiency.
(c) Dermatitis herpetiformis.
(d) Coeliac disease.

144 (a) Narrowing and ulceration of the transverse colon and caecum. It is noteworthy that the hepatic flexure appears normal between these two involved segments of colon (skip lesions).
(b) Crohn's disease.

145 (a) Lichen planus.
(b) Oesophageal ulceration and stricture formation.
(c) A combination of systemic corticosteroids and antisecretory drugs. Oesophageal dilatation should be withheld unless symptoms fail to respond to drug treatment.

146 (a) Infectious mononucleosis.
(b) Treatment of the sore throat with ampicillin.

147 (a) Pseudoxanthoma elasticum.
(b) The retina, which may show angioid streaks.
(c) Vascular degeneration in the gastrointestinal tract.

148 (a) Smooth tongue, angular cheilitis.
(b) Iron-deficiency anaemia.
(c) Rectal examination, testing any stool on the examining glove for the presence of occult blood, sigmoidoscopy and rectal biopsy.

149 (a) Splinter haemorrhages.
(b) Infective endocarditis.
(c) Mesenteric ischaemia, probably due to an arterial embolus.

150 (a) Pneumatic balloon dilatation for achalasia of the cardia.
(b) Oesophageal perforation.

151, 152 (a) Zinc deficiency.
(b) Review of intravenous zinc supplementation, together with rapid resolution following zinc administration.

153 (a) Enterocutaneous fistula.
(b) Sinography may confirm communication with affected bowel.

154 (a) Methaemoglobinaemia leading to cyanosis.
(b) Treatment with dapsone.

155 (a) Scurvy, leading to perifollicular haemorrhages.
(b) The gums may show gingivitis and hypertrophy.
(c) Measurement of leucocyte ascorbic acid concentration.

156 (a) Small bowel enema (enteroclysis).
(b) More rapid filling of small bowel loops than with conventional follow through X-ray, together with the ability to distend the small bowel directly, giving good quality double-contrast views of the mucosa.

157 (a) There is a diminutive polyp.
(b) Because the bowel preparation is poor, *no* attempt should be made to electrocoagulate the polyp at this time because of the explosion risk. This tiny polyp can be biopsied with safety using conventional endoscopic forceps. If it proves to be adenomatous, it may be wise to proceed to formal colonoscopy after full bowel preparation to exclude synchronous neoplasia elsewhere in the colon.

158 (a) Digital subtraction selective coeliac arteriography.
(b) Insulinoma, causing hypoglycaemia with behavioural manifestations.

159 (a) Psoriasis.
(b) Hepatic fibrosis due to methotrexate.

160 (a) Inflammatory bowel disease, especially Crohn's disease.
(b) Erythrocyte sedimentation rate, C-reactive protein, serum albumin, serum B12 and folate, sigmoidoscopy, rectal biopsy, barium enema (or colonoscopy) and barium follow-through (or small bowel enema).

161 (a) Cutting biopsy needle ('Trucut needle').
(b) Percutaneous liver biopsy, biopsy of abdominal masses under ultrasound guidance.

162, 163 (a) Haemobilia (blood clot is protruding from the ampulla and is demonstrated within the opacified biliary tree).
(b) Percutaneous liver biopsy.

164, 165 (a) Amoebic dysentery (one *Entamoeba histolytica* trophozoite with ingested red cell remnants is seen in the centre of the microscopic field).
(b) A five- to ten-day course of oral metronidazole.

166 (a) Two anal fissures.
(b) Straining at constipated stools.

167 (a) Congenital intrinsic duodenal obstruction.
(b) Oesophageal atresia, annular pancreas.

168 (a) Para-oesophageal (rolling) hiatus hernia.
(b) Surgical repair is usually recommended because of the high risk of acute dilatation, perforation or volvulus formation.

169 (a) Aortic bifurcation grafting.
(b) Ischaemic colitis. The inferior mesenteric artery is commonly sacrificed during aortic bifurcation grafting. Ischaemic complications may occur if the collateral arterial supply is inadequate.

170 (a) Secondary syphilis.
(b) Serological tests.

171 (a) Mallory–Weiss tear (mucosal tear).
(b) Repeated vomiting or retching, alcohol over-indulgence.

172 (a) Hereditary angio-oedema.
(b) Demonstration of reduced serum concentrations of C_1 esterase inhibitor.

173 (a) An ulcer of the antrum of the stomach. This is likely to be a benign peptic ulcer.
(b) Treatment of spondylitis with non-steroidal anti-inflammatory drugs.
(c) Malignancy may be excluded by endoscopy and biopsy of the ulcer.

174 (a) Jaundice, pigmentation, blood clot around mouth.
(b) Primary biliary cirrhosis.
(c) Bleeding oesophageal varices.

175 (a) Alcoholic cirrhosis.
(b) Spironolactone (an aldosterone antagonist).

176 (a) Slow release potassium chloride, non-steroidal anti-inflammatory drugs.
(b) Intestinal perforation. Fibrous scar formation around the ulcer may lead to intestinal obstruction.

177 (a) Idiopathic haemochromatosis (note the 'slatey grey' pigmentation).
(b) Weekly venesection until liver iron deposition has been cleared.
(c) Primary hepatocellular carcinoma.

178 (a) Whipple's disease.
(b) Broad spectrum antibiotic therapy. Patients may require supplementation with folic acid, fat soluble vitamins and minerals.

179 (a) Serum auto-antibodies (anti-nuclear antibody, smooth muscle antibody); immunoglobulins; prothrombin time; abdominal ultrasonography.
(b) Wilson's disease—this can mimic chronic active hepatitis, even in the absence of neurological features.

180 (a) The ulcer may be a sign of a more serious disorder, such as Crohn's disease, gastric cancer or lymphoma; the patient may not be complying with drug treatment; or he may have an underlying gastrinoma, causing the Zollinger–Ellison syndrome with gastric acid hypersecretion.
(b) Biopsy of the ulcer, fasting serum gastrin.

181 (a) Behçet's syndrome.
(b) Genital ulceration, involvement of the skin and joints, central nervous system involvement.

182, 183 (a) Macroglossia and signs of trauma from recent tongue-biting.
(b) Amyloidosis (AL subtype).
(c) Multiple myeloma.

Index

Numbers refer not to pages, but to the number shared by the illustration, question and answer.

Notes

Notes

Notes